For Goodness' Sake

For

Goodness'
Sake

*A daily book of cheer
for nurses' aides
and others who care*

Bethany G. Knight, CNA

Foreword by
Janet Budd, CNA

Hartman Publishing

FOR GOODNESS' SAKE: A Daily Book of Cheer
for Nurses' Aides and Others Who Care.

Copy editors: Susan Alvare and Celia McIntire
Cover oil painting: Karen Cole, Santa Fe, NM
Cover and text design: John Cole GRAPHIC DESIGNER,
    Santa Fe, NM

First Printing 1997
Second Revised Printing 1999

ISBN 1-888343-25-7

For information contact:

Hartman Publishing, Inc.
8529-A Indian School Road NE
Albuquerque, NM 87112
(505) 291-1274

I have worked at Countryside Place and Rehabilitation Facility in Mishawalka, Indiana, for 22 years. You could say, it is my only "real job." Before I was selected to be a member of the 1998 National CAN Leadership Council, sponsored by Beverly Healthcare, the only CNAs I knew were the ones I worked with at Countryside. I often wondered, "Does anyone know we exist on this Planet Earth?"

Through my service on the CNALC, I have had an opportunity to meet many loving, caring CNAs from around the country. I have learned that all of us face the same struggles, challenges, and rewards.

My leadership role with the Council also allowed me to meet Bethany Knight, the author of *For Goodness' Sake*. Through her book, I found someone who not only knows we exist, but loves us.

It has been a real inspiration to meet Bethany and read this book. The powerful love she has for all CNAs has helped me to hang in there when I felt I could no longer go on. She has helped me see we are the residents' extended family. We give most residents something to live for, because they know they are loved. The majority of the people on this earth could not do what we chose to do for our elderly. We are God's Angels at work. All CNAs have to stand together and be proud of what we do.

Remember, there isn't a problem that's not solvable in the workplace.

Reading *For Goodness' Sake* has helped me get through many challenges. I keep it at my bedside when I need to be uplifted. If you truly love what you do as a CNA, you will benefit greatly from this book.

Janet Budd, CNA
Countryside Place and
    Rehabilitation Center
Mishawalka, Indiana

In the late 1950's, Roger Greeley, my father, opened the first senior citizen center in Michigan, the 60-Plus Drop In Center. Housed in the basement of the People's Church, the Unitarian Church he served in Kalamazoo for nearly thirty years, 60-Plus was also my after school program. On the laps of the program participants, I was schooled in the wonder of growing old.

My mother, Kay Greeley, volunteered for years as a hospital 'Gray Lady', performing many of the duties of a CNA. Shaped by my parents' example, I was further spoiled by doting grandparents, and early on I became an unabashed lover of the elderly.

Some thirty years after first having cookies with Miss Jean Williams in that basement, I began my career with Vermont nursing homes. For about two years I worked as a long term care ombudsman in the state's nursing and residential care homes. I fielded complaints from facility residents, complaints that almost always boiled down to "I'm lonely. I want to be noticed." In 1986, the Vermont Care Association (VHCA, Vermont's trade organization for these homes) had need of an executive director. A friend told me to apply.

My love for the elderly, coupled with a deep desire for the culture to wake up and revere their presence, inspired me to lead the VHCA for more than 10 years. During this decade, I expanded my love for the elderly to include those who care for them as well.

Between 1989 and 1991, I led 50 workshops for nursing assistants, workshops in which I learned a great deal about the rigors of your work. Each session produced beautiful stories of care. Aides would share tales of hearing fears and confessions, offering comfort at the deathbed, or trying to soothe the tragic consequences of bitter family feuds. Wishing to share these moments of greatness, I began to write this book, as a tribute to the world's most noble profession.

In 1995, at Maple Lane Nursing Home in Barton, VT, I completed training for, and was licensed as, a nursing assistant. I have yet to work a full eight-hour day in this capacity; it is so demanding. More than ever, I came to respect the incredible service of America's nursing assistants.

In 1997, I launched Northern Knights, my own creative services company. My mission has been to awaken CNAs to use their voice, coaching them to speak powerfully about the work. You've always been caring, now it's time to be daring! Traveling the nation, meeting with thousands of CNAs, I have confirmed what I learned in Vermont's nursing and residential care homes—you are modern day saints, a blessing to us all!

Remember, all life will be treasured, and peace will comfort the planet when the caregivers of the world tell their precious love stories. This book contains a few. Make sure you start telling yours.

God bless you all.

Bethany Knight
Glover, Vermont
March 1999

January

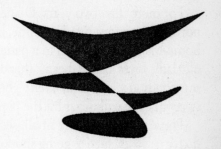

You are one of 1.5 million nurses' aides bathing, dressing, feeding and loving patients twenty-four hours a day in nursing homes across this country.

Unfortunately we only read about you and your work when you make a mistake, as when Ora Lee got her name in the national news. The fifty-six-year-old nurses' aide from Mississippi hit a patient.

For more than two years, Diane, a nurses' aide in a northern Vermont nursing home, has been smuggling home-made baked beans to a patient. Seems the little old lady loves baked beans (her favorite food), but somebody decided they aren't good for her. Diane's sweet gesture will never hit the papers.

Praise yourself for the small, secret things that you do for patients, such as going shopping for their grandson's birthday, fixing their hair a special way, coming in on your day off, or giving away a favorite pin.

We won't read your name in the newspapers—just on your patients' faces.

TODAY: Praise yourself.

In your town, successful people drive brand-new cars that would take more than 250 of your weekly paychecks to buy—almost five years of your pay.

One hour of the muffler installer's services costs you four hours of your pay. When your toilet breaks, you pay five times your hourly wage for help, parts not included.

Television tells you having money means you've made it. The more money you have, the more successful you are. Right?

Wrong! The real test of success is what happens between people, the loving kindnesses that we exchange.

How many people hear "I love you" from the people they work with? How many bankers get kisses and hugs from their customers?

Once you realize your heart is your bank, you'll never feel poor again.

TODAY: Be happy! You're rich!

Most of the old people who end up needing your care are poor women over the age of eighty-five. They have a problem with their bones, bladder and/or brain. Like you, they never made enough money to save for their old age. So the government pays for their care, through Medicaid and Medicare. But these tax dollars don't go far enough.

About 70 cents of every dollar spent in a nursing home is spent on staff wages and benefits. The other 30 cents pays for food, taxes, insurance, electricity, heat, phones, supplies, new furniture, roof repairs and so on.

Your employer is not paid enough by Medicaid and Medicare to pay you what you deserve. That is because this country has not discovered a way to pay for long term healthcare.

So you are underpaid. And until the people of this country, and our government, decide to pay enough for taking care of old people, you will be underpaid.

Being underpaid does not mean it is fair or right. It means you are modern day saints, willing to lovingly care for fragile old people who have no one else to turn to. Thank God for you.

TODAY: Realize you were born before your time.

Being old in America is not much to look forward to. While we all are afraid of death and don't want to die young, we also (strangely enough) are afraid of getting old.

Remember the beauty cream commercial? The actress, who looks about seventeen, is worried about wrinkles and says she is "going to fight aging every step of the way!"

Maybe she should kill herself and declare victory?

Let's not forget all the family members who don't come to visit your patients because they are so uncomfortable with seeing a loved one grow old.

Is it any surprise, then, that you, who have chosen to care for our old treasures, are as devalued as the elderly themselves?

People ask you, "How can you work there? Isn't it depressing? It smells so bad, and people are dying. You must be a special kind of person."

In a way these strangers are right. You are special because you have discovered an ancient truth: love comes in all sizes, shapes, ages and smells. And you get and give some every day.

TODAY: Looking in the mirror, say "I am special!"

Today, pick up a newspaper and go to the classified advertisements at the back.

Now look under the personals column, all the people looking for love.

"Let us give your healthy, white, newborn baby a happy, secure home. Call us collect. Bill and Mary."

"Single white male seeking attractive brunette, age 20–28, for fun, romance and possibly more. Write Bob."

The Cupid Connection, Dating Exchange, Love Partners—everyone is thinking that, to be happy, they need to have their perfect picture of Mister or Miss or Baby Right. Healthy, slim, young. And they also think that, until they have these ideal relationships, their lives will be empty, without love, incomplete.

Invite them to visit you at work! Let them see that you get paid to love, and lead far from an empty life.

TODAY: Share the good news of your work.

Have you ever considered the power you have?

Do you realize that most of the people you work with would not and could not exist without you? No kidding!

Lying in their beds, or slumped in their chairs, they await your arrival. Just going to the bathroom is something they cannot do without you.

They listen for your voice. Why, some know you're coming just by hearing your step! They ask about your family, your evening, your new haircut.

In their little, still lives, you are the scenery that goes by. You are the beautiful view. You are the proof that life goes on.

You, even when you feel overtired, underpaid, short-staffed, hung over, angry, depressed, sick or fed up, are just what they need. In your own way you are perfect.

TODAY: Live up to your greatness.

On those rare occasions your patient has a visitor, have you ever heard any of the conversation?

Usually the visitor talks a bit nervously about life "out there"—work, kids, school. Sometimes they mention how friends are, or stores that have closed. Pets and house renovations are reported upon too.

Often a little gift is brought, such as a plant, flowers, or chocolate. Those times when photographs are shared are especially happy.

After these pleasantries, your patient is asked: "Well, how are you, Mom?" Or Dad, or Gram, or whoever.

They usually say "OK" or "about the same." And then the room gets quiet. It just seems hard to think of other things to say.

Until you enter the room. "Well here's someone I want you to meet!" they say, reaching out for you. What comes next is news of your life, your kids, your dog, your luck.

TODAY: Count your best friends at work.

Caregivers like you almost seem to have the desire to give in their blood.

You usually were the helper at home, taking care of the little kids or helping with Gramma. Growing up, you baby-sat.

Working in a day care, school, group home or other care-setting wouldn't scare you. Your life is about caring for others. How many years have you been a paid caregiver?

Through this caring, you derive great personal satisfaction. Like the old Raggedy Anne doll that says "I love you" on her chest, your heart reads, "I care."

While others jump from job to job, quitting because they hate the work, the boss, and the pay, you have found your place.

You have come to see rewards for taking care of others. You know that in bringing comfort you find comfort, that in loving you are loved.

TODAY: Be satisfied with you.

January 9

Some days are just more exhausting than others. There's no doubt about it, being a nurses' aide is physically and emotionally draining. At the end of the shift, you can be so tired, with an aching back and pounding head. Some days you can feel your heart beating in your calves.

Days off are not only fun, they are critical. Without them, you can't recharge your own batteries and prepare yourself for the next hard day at work. Your mind and body need to rest, to have some quiet, a change of pace.

Cherish your days off. Use them wisely. Yes, to get the laundry and shopping done, but also to catch up on your soaps, have coffee with a friend, call your mom.

Or just to sit outdoors and feel the sun and breeze on your skin.

Remember, your first responsibility is to take care of yourself. Then you can take care of others.

TODAY: Be good to you.

When you neglect you, everyone suffers

So they asked you to work on your day off, and you said yes. Or a double shift, and you said yes.

Now, when you're beat, you're angry and ready to blame. Remember, you said yes. There's no victim here—except perhaps your patient, who doesn't deserve your crankiness.

Being responsible for your life means making decisions in your best interest. Saying yes when you mean no doesn't serve anyone well. Instead it simply assures you a trip into the land of resentment.

If you're asked to work extra and you don't want to, say so. Tell your supervisor you understand the pinch everyone is in, but that you know yourself and you need a day off. Rather than thinking you don't care, let them know that it is because you do care that you are going to take this needed break. Then, when you come back to work, you'll be refreshed and ready to give again.

TODAY: Be responsible for your well-being.

Do you feel guilty when you choose something for yourself? Or ask others to do something for themselves?

Caregivers are notoriously co-dependent personalities—men and women who can never seem to think of themselves first or think of themselves without thinking of others.

Yes, a great sense of personal worth comes with taking care of others, of being needed. But if this feeling is not balanced by a desire for the other person or patient to take some responsibility, trouble can occur.

Just as you need to feel needed and strong, so does your patient. Encourage her to do what is possible for herself, even if it is not as swift or smooth as you would like. Help her experience some of her own ability and independence again.

Healthy relationships are interdependent ones, where people see themselves as separate and able.

TODAY: Let go when you need to.

Looking back over our lives, certain loving people shine forth.

Who is the most caring person you have ever known?

For some of us the answer to this question comes fast and easy. Oh, my mother, of course. My grandmother. My sister. My husband.

For others, we need to think awhile. Was it a teacher? Someone we worked with? Could it be another nurses' aide?

Take some time to answer this question, identifying for yourself what it was that made the person you would choose so caring. What about them impressed you? How did they express their caring heart? How did they make you feel?

Once you know who your most caring person is, make sure you let them know your feelings. Even if they are no longer nearby, or even if they are dead, say a silent prayer of thanks.

Then take a moment to consider that, in some way, you resemble this caring person. Let it sink in that, in choosing this person as your model or standard, you resemble them. We admire people we wish to be like.

TODAY: Whom do you resemble?

Bingo, bowling, shopping, dancing, partying, being with our friends and families—each of us has our own idea of fun.

Nurses' aides who love their jobs know that, sometimes, work can be more fun than play.

Think of those funny moments when a confused patient accused you of something so outrageous that all you could do was laugh? Or when another aide took an angry, combative patient and danced the Texas two-step with him until he relaxed?

Life in a nursing home is just that. Life. It is no different than the world outside the window. The community is smaller and the relationships are more defined, but the possibilities for joy and closeness are just as great.

For the patients, this institution, right now, is their home. No one needs to hold back laughter or love for another time or place. This is it; they must live every day as fully as they can, for each day may well be their last.

TODAY: Have fun at work.

To a small child or a dog everybody is the same.

Kids and pets don't see some people as patients and others as nurses' aides. They treat everyone the same. For kids, every person is a lap, someone to play with. For dogs, everyone is a potential bearer of treats!

Some days at work we can forget how much we all have in common, how few differences really exist. We all want to be respected, liked, secure, safe, needed.

In the rush of the shift, it is easy to forget that our coworkers are often as hungry for kindness as our patients. Who knows what kind of argument or pain they left at home today? Being only human, it is easy to impatiently judge others when they are cross or grouchy. We usually say "Carol is such a snot today!" instead of "I wonder why Carol is so upset?"

Reminding ourselves that no one wants to have a bad day, we can reach out with tenderness and understanding. We can offer our care and healing power to patients and coworkers.

TODAY: Bring love and cheer to other aides.

Having known the sting of gossip, one would think we would all retire from the sport, since the injuries are so great.

But we keep on whispering and tattling, finding some perverse intimacy and pleasure with others.

At mealtime and breaks in some healthcare facilities the unwritten request would seem to be "please pass the bad news." Marge and Sandy like to talk about Gloria. Cruel, catty stories about Gloria become the sleazy basis for Marge and Sandy's friendship. They feel closer, but in truth they are more alone than ever.

Marge and Sandy will never fully trust each other because they will always fear being turned upon. And of course, any chance for a friendship with Gloria is hopeless.

The only sure cement for real friendships is love.

Closeness comes from sharing our own lives, not dissecting the lives of others. While it is more risky to talk about ourselves, it is more honest.

TODAY: Repeat no gossip.

Bad days at work are as common as head colds—and just as contagious. The causes of both are mysterious; the only cure is the passing of time.

Young nurses' aide James T. had been on the job in a 120-patient nursing home for more than a year when he began to think seriously about what makes a bad day.

"Some days," he explained, "I would go home and feel just awful, just rotten, as though I wanted to quit. Then, other days, I would go home and feel great, as though it was the best day of my life. And I couldn't see what made the difference."

One afternoon during a staff in-service training workshop, James found himself listening to other aides describe a bad day.

All of a sudden James stood up with the look of pure delight, a man ready to report a discovery.

"I know why I have good days and bad days!" he declared. "A good day is when I spend my time thinking of the patients, what they need, how they feel. A bad day happens when I spend my time thinking of myself, feeling sorry for me."

TODAY: Keep your heart and mind on others.

The more advances in medical science, the longer we live. And the longer we live, the greater our chances of having some form of dementia or senility.

National statistics suggest that up to 60 percent of patients in an average nursing home have some form of mental disorder. That makes the job of the caregiver even tougher.

Gone are the days of simply making sure an alert patient is well fed, clean and dry. Nurses' aides now must try to figure out the needs of patients who are unable to communicate or cooperate. Many patients don't even know where they are.

Caring for agitated, disturbed old people, you can feel pretty unappreciated. The words "thank you" are as rare as they are in a preschool. Like an untrained child, the dementia patient doesn't know.

If possible, ask the family members to tell you about the patients' personalities before they got so ill. Ask for photos of them in their robust days. Keep favorite stories about them in the front of your mind while you give them personal care.

TODAY: Take care of the person, not their disability.

Demented patients are often violent patients. Confused as to where they are and who is trying to do what to them, they feel attacked. Their instincts tell them to protect and defend themselves.

Such is the illogical logic that drives Ernie to smack you in the face when you prepare him for his shower. Or the reason Bea rakes her jagged nails down your arm at bedtime. Or why Louise spits and kicks when its time for her medicine.

Sure, your training warned you plenty about not hurting the patients. But no one mentioned what to do when you are abused. It sure is hard to keep your cool when your glasses have just been knocked off.

And it's even harder to go back to Ernie's bedside the next day, knowing what just might happen. For Violette L., a nurses' aide for twenty-three years, the hardest part of her work is not just going back the next day. "The hardest part of my job is to forgive the patient who has hurt me, to go back and give him a hug."

TODAY: Forgive your attackers and begin again—with love.

When speech goes, we humans feel pretty lost.

Stroke, Alzheimer's, paralysis and mouth cancer leave many patients with limited or no communication skills. They sit, sometimes drooling onto their shirts, unable to express their wishes.

Those of us who have raised children know that, by paying careful attention to our babies, we could often figure out what they needed. A certain cry meant hunger; another whine meant wet diaper.

Betty decided to use these same detective skills with Evelyn, a patient who had suffered five strokes. "Whenever I went into Evelyn's room, she would bug her eyes out and make a loud 'oo-oo-oo' noise," recalled Betty. "She sounded mad, and I was afraid to take care of her."

One day Betty made a decision. A great deal of Evelyn's brain was dead, killed off by a devastating stroke. Evelyn's 'oo-oo-oo' noise was one of the few forms of self-expression Evelyn had left.

"I decided that when Evelyn said 'oo-oo-oo' it meant 'How are you?" said Betty. With this nice thought in mind, Betty created a whole new attitude for delivering Evelyn's care.

TODAY: Assign loving meanings to unusual behaviors.

The next time you're in McDonald's notice how the staff has been trained to give a particular response.

Whenever one worker makes a request such as "I need two fries and a coffee" to a fellow worker, the other crew member always responds with "thank you."

The "thank you" serves as confirmation that the order got through, that the kitchen will prepare two servings of French fries and a coffee. But it also puts kind words into the atmosphere on a regular basis.

Working on a wing or a shift where there is a lot of complaining and anger, the air gets pretty polluted with foul energy. It's like being in a factory town: When thick black clouds are belched into the air, things get pretty dark. It's hard to look on the bright side when everyone's mood is so gloomy.

Saying thank you, bless you, have a nice day, and other such friendly phrases, can make work a much sunnier place. Supervisors aren't the only employees who can say, "You did a nice job!" Feel free to pump out good words and thoughts whenever you want.

TODAY: Sprinkle kind words throughout your day.

The loyalty some people feel for certain baseball teams, makes of cars and kinds of soda can be pretty incredible.

Don't tell a Red Sox fan that the Montreal Expos are just as good, or suggest to a Toyota driver that your Chevy is better. And be warned right now that serving Coke to a Pepsi drinker is grounds for abandonment!

Our nature is to stake our claim, deciding what is ours and getting pretty territorial about it. Seniors hang out with seniors, juniors with juniors. And the freshmen! They had better stay away.

In a healthcare facility, such loyalty can go too far and turn into turf wars. The second shift is convinced the entire third shift is lazy. B wing believes A wing has it easy. And all the aides think the nurses are just plain useless.

In such a combat zone the patients suffer most. Staff energy is devoted to silly squabbles, and the environment gets more and more hostile. When you reach this battle stage it's time to send out negotiators. Volunteer to work with the group you are having the most trouble with, or transfer to another shift or wing. Quickly show yourself and everyone that nothing is more important than quality care for patients. Remind each other that your loyalty is to your work first.

TODAY: Make peace, not war.

We who live in northern climates are deep into winter today—beautiful white snow, delicate window pane frost, sparkling icicles hanging from the porch roof.

Oh yes, we mustn't forget the dead car batteries, below-zero mornings and ice-covered roads!

How we miss the sun, warm and welcoming. Some of us even suffer from an actual disease, Seasonal Affective Disorder (SAD), that makes us sad and depressed with so little sunlight.

We had a good time decorating the building for Christmas and enjoying all the goodies. Now, less than a month later, we are down in the dumps.

Is today a good day to wear your silly purple telephone earrings? Or your rainbow colored suspenders? Or the stockings with little watermelons on them?

Everybody needs some colorful moments to improve their moods. And if you are feeling blue or blah, you can imagine your patients are even more down.

TODAY: Be a surprise package!

No one knows what a daily routine is better than a dairy farmer does—up before dawn, feed and milk the cows, 365 days a year.

Some of us thrive on routine. The more predictable our day, the better we feel. We like to know our coffee break is at ten o'clock and that our patients get their hair done the second and fourth Friday of the month.

Others of us like the spice of variety. We like meeting a new patient, learning a new skill, being asked to work in the kitchen at breakfast.

Our patients are just as particular and opinionated. Some like the same aide to dress them every morning at the same time and feed them the same breakfast. Others like the excitement of a new aide bringing them a homemade Finnish *riisipiirika!*

The good news is that all types of staff and patients are needed in your institution. Such differences bring balance to the building, allowing many ideas to be presented and tried.

Rather than judge and criticize someone who does things in a style the opposite of yours, why not celebrate your individuality? *Vive la différence.* How lucky you are to work where you can have your own style.

TODAY: See different ways that work.

When to step outside of the pattern and when not to, that is the question.

Clearly there are certain personal care and medical procedures that you must follow exactly. Lifting, for example, if not done properly, can result in serious injury to you and your patient.

But aren't there times when you don't have to be a robot, a creature of habit?

The change of shift in a nursing home can be a chaotic, noisy time. Studies have shown that more patients fall and are injured around shift time that any other time. Is it because the staff is looking more at the time clock than the stairways?

Rather than rushing out at exactly seven, three or eleven, stop and talk with the lady at the end of the hall who always wants to talk when you're in a rush. Or drop by the kitchen and tell the cook how many people liked her (or his) coffeecake this morning.

Giving yourself an extra five minutes may shake up a few folks ("It's three o'clock! What are you doing?") and that's okay. You can start a trend all by yourself. You control your own schedule, and, once your shift is over, you alone decide when you're ready to go out the door.

TODAY: Take time saying goodbye.

It's amazing what is and isn't written in your job description.

In some facilities nurses' aides work as if the entire well-being of the building and all the patients were their responsibility. They observe everybody's every move, commenting throughout the day on who does and says what.

Other aides are more like Theresa R., a woman I met one day about 3:15 p.m. on my way to a meeting in her facility. Theresa was carrying a large bucket of ice down the stairs, and she was struggling.

"Where are you headed with that?" I asked, wondering why ice would be needed at this time of the afternoon.

"Oh, I like to get things set up for the girls at night," she smiled shyly. "It's for their juices."

No supervisor or job description in the world could have made Theresa haul that ice down from the kitchen after her shift had ended. That loving act was dictated by something deep inside her beautiful heart, something that fueled her sweet smile and caring eyes.

TODAY: Be you.

When you've got forty-eight patients to put to bed and three aides show up, you start behind. No matter what you do, you're behind before you begin.

The hot August night I witnessed this very situation, I began to see how tremendously frustrating an aide's job can be. You want to take good care of each patient and make sure everybody has time on the toilet and maybe even a little back rub. But you can't slow the clock!

Experienced aides—I call them the kings and queens—know how to handle these times. Veterans of many such impossible mornings and evenings, they have learned to just do the best they can. They don't let the obvious frazzle them. Somehow everything will get done, everyone will get taken care of, the day will end.

Like calm mothers with colicky babies, old-timer aides know the worst thing they can do is get nervous, upset and freaked out. By staying even-tempered they truly minister to their patients, sparing them the anxiety. Senior varsity players on your care team, these aides remind us that external circumstances don't dictate their performance. Their personal commitment to kindness is what counts. No matter what.

TODAY: Find a king or queen aide to model.

When you call in sick, but you're not, everybody knows.

As much as we like to think it is okay, or for a good reason, calling in sick when you're not is lying.

So is claiming you're injured when you're not.

Besides the legal and professional consequences (you could be fired if found out) what do such actions do to you?

First and foremost they reduce the value of your word with others. People begin to discount what you say, as if they can't quite trust or believe you any more. "Is her daughter really that sick?" they wonder.

Your word and your actions are all that really matter. What you promise but don't deliver doesn't count. Where you live, what you drive or wear are equally unimportant. What you say and do determines whether you have real friends—and their respect—or not.

Beyond what others think, lying is hazardous to your own health. You do damage to what you think of yourself when you lie. When you need to lie to get your way, it means you haven't yet figured out how to use your personal power appropriately.

TODAY: Tell the truth.

Plenty of magazines seem to print plenty of articles about commitment. Headlines mention men being committed to women, women to men. Seems harder and harder for people to make a commitment.

Look around you. Notice how many of us have ex-husbands and ex-wives. Former roommates and bosses. We're so easily dissatisfied and ready to call it quits, to move on.

That's why meeting Helen and Amy was such an amazing moment for me.

It was a humid Friday afternoon in late May. Sitting with a group of nurses' aides in a tiny home (only thirty patients), I asked how many years they had worked as aides.

Helen had to consult with Amy. "We started in the old building the same year. Was that thirty-two or thirty-five years ago?"

Shazam! There were aides in the room who hadn't combed their own hair or buttered their own toast that long!

What was even more astounding than their decades of service was the commitment behind the years. Their work-life was no different from yours—difficult patients, low wages, unfair supervisors. Yet Amy and Helen had stuck with the job. These two lovely women had made a commitment and had lived up to it.

TODAY: Tell someone about your commitment to work.

My husband teases me, but I think I'm right.

When I see a man with long nose hairs, I wonder about the condition of his marriage. For me, being a good wife includes making sure my husband looks well-groomed. So I trim his nose hairs.

What kind of impression do you create about your place of work? Do your friends only know the problems? Do you share the special stories of cherished patients? Do you describe the hugs you give and receive?

Overhearing women talk in the grocery store, I cringe sometimes about what is said publicly. "That charge nurse is such a _____" or "I asked for the day off, and do you know what he said?"

To make our buildings the best places to live and work, we need to recruit good fellow employees. With halls full of loving, caring nurses' aides, any facility can be transformed overnight. But as the old saying goes, you can draw more flies with honey than with vinegar.

Referring to our work, we need to speak about the good things, the high points. We need to educate others about the pleasures of caring for the elderly and ill.

TODAY: Sing your job's praises!

Before Mother Teresa died, she had been trying to retire from her post as head of the Missionaries of Charity for several years. As the founder of this international religious order, Mother Teresa, like her sisters, ministered to the poorest and dirtiest of the world.

Despite her desire to step down as head mother, the nuns kept reelecting her to the position. Her identity was so closely linked to this famous order, that Mother Teresa became a symbol of pure, selfless love.

If your coworkers were to appoint you to a position in the building, what would it be? What does your style or personality represent?

Are you the funny one? The mothering one? The patient one?

Or are you the cross one? The depressed one? The always sick one?

Think a little longer about this imaginary position of honor. What would your patients say? How do they see you?

TODAY: What's your official title?

A retired nurse who worked most of her years in the maternity ward of a rural hospital told me she was certain that more babies were born on the full moon than at any other time.

While my experience with childbirth is limited to my one son, Elliot (whose birthday is today! Happy birthday, honey!), I like the full moon theory. After all, Elliot was three weeks overdue and finally arrived with the full moon.

Who's to say what unseen forces may be affecting our minds and bodies? Why do deaths in nursing homes seem to be cyclical, with a rise during the Christmas season? Some say patients can't bear the thought of being alone on this major holiday, so they just let go.

Hospital admissions of terminally ill patients seem to go up just before Christmas too.

Often a patient will live just to her birthday, anniversary, or other important date, and then suddenly die. Reaching a personal milestone may allow our patients to spiritually settle in a peaceful fashion. With a tender memory close by, they can leave this world.

TODAY: Be sensitive to special dates.

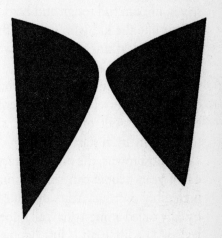

A new month! It's a perfect time for giving yourself and others a fresh start. If you're like most of us, the New Year's resolutions you made just thirty-two days ago have long been forgotten. It just seemed too hard to make changes, didn't it?

Quitting smoking, being more patient, losing weight, or wrestling down the addiction alligator are never easy. In fact, when we work to improve ourselves, life can feel tough and hard.

But like the kid who falls for the hundredth time when she's learning to ice skate, we just need to keep the faith and try again.

What have you disappointed yourself about? When did you let yourself down? Rather than pouring your energy into guilt or, worse yet, self-hatred, declare today your "fresh start day."

In most towns, the public library declares that, one day a year, people can return library books that are incredibly overdue. Years overdue. And on that day, usually called amnesty day, all is forgiven. No fines are levied. The librarian is just happy to have the books back in circulation.

Put your guilt and disappointment on the shelf and get back into circulation. Today is a grand day to begin again.

TODAY: Make a fresh start.

So the big question this morning is, "Did the ground-hog see his shadow?"

As one of the special events for the superstitious, old Punxsutawny Phil's appearance can make or break our winter blahs. And he's not the only creature who triggers our moods and attitudes.

Some of us truly believe that black cats in our paths, a four leaf clover in the front yard, or even finding a dime in the pay phone can signal a change in our luck.

Have some fun at work today. Tell a grumpy aide that you read palms. Take a look at her tired, worn hand, and tell her today is going to be a great day. Or tell a sad aide that, seeing how the milk she poured into her coffee was hardly cloudy, you're certain sunny days are coming.

The Eskimos living at Rocky Point, Alaska, a hundred years ago believed a tingling big toe meant good fortune was coming. Ask your patients if they have any special signs or signals they believe in. You just might hear a great old story.

TODAY: Your smile is a sure sign of a good day.

Living with a lot of people is never easy. Remember all the silly rules you lived with at school? One kid in the bathroom at a time? Line up by height, tallest kid last?

All of these regulations were created to make school life more manageable. And you didn't even stay overnight there!

Nursing homes develop policies and procedures for the same reasons your old principal and teachers did—institutional life is stressful. So many people, so little space.

Jolene, an aide at a nursing home for veterans, was full of complaints about the huge place where she worked. She couldn't understand or accept many of the house rules. Yet she was careful not to let her frustrations affect patient care. "There are some things I don't like at the nursing home," she said, "but none have to do with my people."

This distinction is critical. Your patients didn't write the rules. To be honest, they might dislike things more than you do. But these hassles need not have any influence on your job performance or relationships with needy patients.

Just like school, you can make plenty of friends and have lots of fun in spite of the rules. But please, no food fights, okay?

TODAY: Pay attention to people, not place.

We all have our limits, those invisible lines that nobody had better cross, those beliefs that we won't let go of or compromise.

Aides with very strong opinions have no trouble making themselves known. Shy staff may let thoughts boil inside, never telling a soul.

Patients are the same way. Some folks don't let a moment pass without registering their views, from the burned taste of the cold toast to the noisy television across the hall.

Part of your job is simply to listen to people when they reach their limits, taking some time to hear them out. Often all a person wants is a sympathetic ear, a shoulder to cry on.

But other times, and this is where your judgment comes in, the problem is a real one. Their story is not one you can forget or brush off. Rather, it is something that calls you into action.

When your patient tells you the maintenance man came into her room when she was dressing, you need to make sure her voice is heard. The charge nurse or director of nursing needs to be alerted to this violation of privacy. Matters of privacy, rights, dignity and quality care cannot be ignored.

TODAY: Know when to report real problems.

Who sets policies? In national government, the Congress calls the shots. In the states, the Legislature passes the laws.

In your nursing home, the responsibility isn't as simply or centrally based. While some may think the owner or administrator makes all the decisions, the truth is that good staff can have tremendous clout.

Aides in one home noticed how much the patients seemed to perk up when around bright colors. Neon headbands and colorful earrings always brought comments from patients. One day, when all the white bedspreads were in the laundry, a sunshine yellow spread was put on a bed. The patient couldn't stop exclaiming how "pretty" it was.

With this evidence, the aides went to the administrator and talked to her about needing to make sure the facility used lots of colors. Today, the works of local artists hang in the halls.

How the color story was told made a big difference. Aides didn't storm the administrator's office and say, "Hey, dummy, don't you realize how stupid it is to not use colors here?" How we share our ideas makes or breaks our chances.

Senators and representatives know that even a great idea won't automatically become law. To successfully lobby for change, convincing facts and a persuasive presentation are important. Assume the boss doesn't know yet, not that he or she is stupid, mean, insensitive or purposely avoiding something.

TODAY: Share the responsibility for facility policies.

Children are funny. They go somewhere with you and come away with the oddest impressions and recollections. "Mom, remember when we went to that white house and they had a dog that couldn't go in the kitchen?"

It turns out your son is remembering his first visit to your great uncle's house, where you watched slides of a hunting trip to northern Canada and ate deer and bear meat for dinner. And your five-year-old remembered the dog!

As we grow up, we gradually begin to distinguish what is important and what isn't, what is the wheat and what is the chaff.

It's easy to get so wrapped up in the politics and problems of the job that we forget the point. Some people get so obsessed with money that everything that happens becomes an opportunity to complain about money. An autopsy has been ordered for a dead welfare patient. "Oh great!" the money-minded employee says. "Who's gonna pay for that? Us taxpayers!"

The point of working in a nursing home is to provide care for frail old people in the most loving way possible. That's all. And that's plenty.

TODAY: Ignore the chaff.

Getting married, I was thrilled about having a home with my husband. Being able to go places as a couple and even to wash a man's clothes was exciting.

One of the tiny little ways married life fit me so well involved my wallet. For years, I had walked around worried about who to list on the identification card where it said, "In case of emergency call _____." At last I had a husband to mention!

For your patients, you are often the one and only person they can call. Family are so far away, busy and, in some cases, dead. After all, many eighty-five-year-old women outlive their sixty-five-year-old sons who have heart disease.

A large part of being a caregiver is to regularly deliver assurance. "Everything is okay," you tell them. "Don't worry now, there is always someone here, night and day, to take care of you."

Some of your patients have been alone for a long time. Even before they entered the nursing home, they were all alone in their little house or apartment, maybe getting a plant on Mother's Day, maybe not.

As incredible as it seems, their good old days may be right now. They have never received so much attention from so many kind people before. Your presence is not just about comfort, it is about life, friendship, conversation.

TODAY: Give plenty of reassurances.

Some days, we don't want to be around another living thing. Well, maybe we can stand our cat. But there is no way we want to answer the phone or talk to anybody.

For patients in nursing homes, there is no room for days like these. Whether they like it or not, whether they feel like getting up and dressed or not, or having breakfast or not, you are told to get them up, dressed and fed.

For all you know, one of your ladies spent one weekend a month her whole life in her pajamas, squirreled away in her bedroom with a mystery paperback, with the world locked out. But now you are told to get her up. She might not be able to tell you in words why she resists your help, but her eyes give you a hint.

Or there is the man you take care of who doesn't feel like talking or going to activities. He was a logger and he liked the privacy of the outdoors. By nature he is a loner, a loner who today finds it nearly impossible to share a bedroom with a stranger who keeps trying to talk to him.

Yes, you are just trying to do your job, motivated by the old "suit up and show up" mentality. Unfortunately for everyone involved, some patients are not made for the glaring lights and group experience of a nursing home. They are individuals, people who have marched to a different drummer all their lives.

TODAY: Respect the individuals in your care.

Taking care of difficult patients is just that—difficult. Many aides have found that dealing with patients called "combative" led to serious injury, disability and time away from work. One aide I met was out of work for more than a year following three cosmetic surgeries on her arm—a patient bit her.

During an open discussion, one afternoon, with a group of aides, we got around to the subject of tough patients who can make you want hazardous duty pay. Aides described some pretty awful situations, including dislocated shoulders, broken eyeglasses and verbal threats.

"I wish she would just hit me and get it over with," said one aide, maintaining that the emotional abuse of a patient with a nasty tongue was just as upsetting as physical attacks.

"We would be charged with a crime if we hurt them," another aide said.

Our conversation closed with some thoughts that sounded very wise to all of us. "They don't even know what they are doing. They probably feel like prisoners. If they knew what they were doing, they would be so embarrassed," said a red-headed aide.

Michelle, one of the more angry aides when we began talking about staff abuse, looked around the room. "I've taken this way too personally. I now see they are not here to test me. They're just here."

TODAY: Take no pain personally.

Everybody has some prejudices.

Depending on who raised you and where you lived, you may feel uncomfortable with people of different colors, with southern accents or Catholics.

When healthcare workers get dressed for work, just as we put our shoes on, we need to consciously take off our prejudices and leave them at home. Like dark glasses that filter our vision, prejudice distorts what we see.

One of the greatest temptations when working in a healthcare facility is to judge our patients. "He wouldn't have to be here if he hadn't had so much booze that he pickled his liver." "She's so fat, no wonder she can't walk!"

Worse yet are the remarks we make to each other about a patient's disease, as if they are lower than us. AIDS patients are acutely aware of prejudiced views and treatment.

To everyone's benefit, our job doesn't require us to have an opinion about patients' problems. In fact, professional caregivers do not pass judgment, but simply deliver good care. To them it matters not how someone became ill and needs care now. What matters is that their patients are trusting them with their lives and they expect the highest standards of unbiased performance.

TODAY: Free yourself of all judgments about patients.

In the 1920s an American woman toured Egypt. Part of the trip included a visit to the ancient tombs. Standing beside a centuries-old mummy, the tourist removed some dry seeds clenched in the mummy's hand.

Back home in the United States, the woman planted the seeds. To her delight, she soon had morning glories.

Who would have ever imagined such a rare occurrence? A very, very old seed, hidden from view, is put in the right environment—and bingo! It surprises all with its lively beauty.

Around you, every day, are old, fragile, often dried up old people. Hidden from the view of their communities, they sit silently, rarely noticed.

Can you create a nursing home environment that causes them to bloom? A place that is so loving, safe and warm that they show their own inner beauty? Look around you. What do you need to do to make your home a greenhouse for people?

Each patient is a potential morning glory. Totally confused dementia patients can surprise you with their flawless ability to harmonize; they just need to be invited to sing. That restless patient who wakes at 3 a.m. every day used to make the donuts at the bakery. Bring him into the kitchen today to enjoy the familiar sounds and smells.

TODAY: Create a home where patients blossom.

Abraham Lincoln was born today. So was I. As a kid, I loved the fact that my birthday was in red on the big black and white calendar that hung in the classroom. Today, those red numbers are no longer. People more powerful than I created "Presidents' Day," and we now celebrate Abe and George's day as one.

President Lincoln is remembered for many things, but none more famous than his "Gettysburg Address," in which he said this country was "of, by and for the people."

How much is your facility "for the people," and how much must the people be "for the facility"? A good way to test yourself is to look at facility flexibility.

Can patients say "no" when they want? Can they choose what outfit they want to wear, or does someone else pick out their clothes?

In computer terminology, people ask if a system is "user friendly," if it is easy for the person to work with it. Is your facility "user friendly"? Are senile patients who want to help the cleaning lady allowed to putter a little bit, or are they crossly pulled from the housekeeper's cart and sent to their rooms? Can patients safely walk around outside and enjoy the healing feeling of the outdoors?

TODAY: Make life easy for your patients.

Dressing for comfort instead of for style is wonderful, isn't it?

On days off, who doesn't put on their grungiest old sweats and a T-shirt, or those jeans that are permanently shaped to your belly and bottom? Living in a nursing home, most residents dress for comfort seven days a week. The sweat suit often becomes the facility uniform for both men and women.

Perhaps this plain wardrobe is one of the reasons that the Cotillion Ball is such a hit at the Mayo Nursing Home in Northfield. The brainchild of administrator Lorraine Day, the ball guarantees Mayo residents one night of sheer elegance. The evening starts with the selection of gowns for the ladies and nice ties and suitcoats for the gentlemen. Collected here and there, the home has a large assortment of real dress-up clothes.

Cotillion invitees don't enter unescorted. In full dress blues, the cadets of Norwich University, the nation's oldest military college, accompany the honored guests. With swords raised, some cadets create a corridor for the grand entry, while others push the wheelchairs through.

Gay streamers and decorations festoon the dining room; there are plenty of hearts and flowers. Staff work as waitresses that night, with boiled shrimp, chocolates and other delectables on the menu. Dancing to a live band follows, and, of course, the champagne flows.

A far cry from sweat suits!

TODAY: Plan some glamour.

Growing up, one of the best holidays at school was Valentine's Day. Pure sweets: candy, cookies, cake, cupcakes, red punch. All those red cinnamon hearts to burn our tongues and massage our hearts with short goofy sayings: Be Mine, Coax Me, Hot Lips.

We carefully decorated big construction paper envelopes, taped them to the fronts of our desks, and waited for the other kids to make their valentine deliveries. In the early grades everybody exchanged cute valentines with cartoon animals and red hearts. As we got older, boys didn't give many, and certainly not to any girls they really liked.

Nursing homes usually do an award-winning job of decorating for Valentine's Day. Even the diabetics seem to get a few candy hearts on their trays. Sometimes children from the school or day care bring by some handmade valentines.

But the valentines most worth receiving are those that aren't made of paper or candy. The real ones aren't labeled or in envelopes. Rather, they are the ones that are found, like the hidden pictures in the old Highlights magazine drawings. The real ones are the looks, the smiles, the hugs, the little squeezes and touches that come when you least expect them.

Gwen, an aide at a 140-patient home, said the best part of the job is when "a patient asks my name." Gwen knows she is loved when that happens. And she knows her patient feels loved, too.

TODAY: Look for hidden valentines.

A characteristic of human beings is that we worry. The Bible warns us not to bother about tomorrow's worries today: "Sufficient unto the day is the evil thereof" (Matthew 6:34). Still, we worry.

Living in a nursing home, everything is taken care of for patients. Meals are planned, cooked and served. Dishes, clothes, sheets and floors are washed. Social and religious activities are planned; medication is given. When needed, assistance is provided for dressing, bathing and using the toilet.

One could think that with so little responsibility, and so much help, a patient could finally stop worrying. One would imagine that the life of a person in a nursing home could be worry free.

As any aide knows, this is far from the case. Many patients, even those who are very confused, will say with a worried look to an aide at lunch, "Waitress, how will I pay for this meal?" Others, who are mentally very alert, will confide anxiously that their savings account is getting small and they don't know how much longer they can pay for their care.

A well-rounded care plan means that all of the patient's needs are considered. We can never fully and totally meet every need, but we can be aware and try our best. Caring for the worried, anxious patient means listening and comforting.

TODAY: Soothe a worried brow.

Several years ago, a grisly story appeared in newspapers across the country. It seems a California woman who owned a board and care home was systematically killing the old patients, burying them in the backyard and collecting their monthly Social Security checks.

Public reaction to the story was intense and singular. "How could she do that? She must be crazy!"

Yes, she had to be crazy. But if we fully consider the crime, it seems the matron had many accomplices. Who? Us. All of us. All of the neighbors, citizens and community residents who didn't miss the murdered people.

Where was the general public's responsibility for the frail, most vulnerable members of the society? To think people could be killed, their checks continued to be delivered, and no one noticed they were gone.

While government inspectors and regulators are regular visitors to nursing homes, sometimes the delivery people are the only real guests. That makes the aide's job even more essential. You are the conscience for the facility, too. Is there anything going on that you don't believe is fair or legal? Would it be smart to review your concerns with your supervisor?

You see situations that no one else witnesses. Don't be afraid to seek advice.

TODAY: Be a wise watchdog.

Someone once said no job is as hard as being a nurses' aide, with the possible exceptions of being a mother and a coal miner. The mother, because you can't quit. The coal miner, because the ceiling could collapse at any moment and you're dead.

Still, being a nurses' aide demands a tremendous range of qualities and skills. Patience, kindness, a sense of humor and fairness, physical and emotional strength, gentleness, efficiency, organizational abilities, and medical knowledge are just a few of the necessary ingredients.

Working as a team, aides quickly see their fellow workers' strengths and weaknesses. No compliment is more meaningful than the praise of one aide for another.

Similarly, no one sees an inferior performance faster than another aide. It's pretty easy to see poor attitude and poor care, and almost always long before the supervisor catches on.

Poor work as an aide doesn't mean the person is a bad person. It simply means they need to improve their approach or they shouldn't be an aide. Perhaps they could star in a totally different line of work.

Waiting for a supervisor to notice a poor performance is not smart. As a professional, your responsibility is to the patient and to quality care.

TODAY: Speak to fellow aides who need coaching.

Sherrie was a pretty tough lady. Clean and sober for six years, she told us a little about her three-generation family of alcoholics.

"One of my fondest memories is sitting on my daddy's lap swigging beer out of his bottle," she said quite seriously.

At 15, she was behind the barn, smoking pot. Not long after that, she began her years of blackout. Sherrie has truly no memories of many, many years. She supported herself working on dairy farms, taking care of cows. "Cows didn't talk back," she explained.

Once she took control of her life, Sherrie began to think about being a nurses' aide. "I wanted to leave farming, but I just didn't think I could face all the nasty cleaning up, you know." A woman who had survived her family, her addictions, and her pain, was stopped by the thought of a bedpan.

An aide now for more than a year, Sherrie laughed at her old fears. "Little messes are so irrelevant," she said, "because I care so much about the people!"

TODAY: Make messes irrelevant.

Gertrude was dying. Everyone could tell. The doctor couldn't do any more; all he told the staff was to keep her comfortable.

To anyone who would listen, Gertrude kept saying "I want my family to visit. I want to see them."

But, though many relatives lived in town, no one came.

Janet, a nurses' aide who also worked as a dietary aide, knew about Gertrude's family. "They haven't spoken to each other in six years, and they are afraid they will run into each other in Gertrude's room. So no one will visit."

With this awareness, Janet made an above-and-beyond the call of duty effort to spend time with Gertrude, comforting her. "I'm here, Gertrude, " Janet would remind her. "I love you."

TODAY: Let no one feel alone.

One thing you can count on as surely as your kids losing the scissors and scotch tape—in every nursing home bathroom there are reminders to "wash your hands!"

And not just after you've been to the bathroom. After you've done personal care, after you've touched dirty laundry, after, it seems, every move you make, you're supposed to wash your hands.

Sometimes we skip that requirement, figuring we know better.

A sanitation inspector once told me of a study he conducted in a midwestern sausage factory. It seemed the bacteria count was pretty high in the links and patties, and he was hired to find out why.

Sitting outside the women's bathroom, he asked each exiting employee, "Did you wash your hands?"

One big lady walked out, listened to his question, and in a defiant tone answered with a loud "NO!"

"Why?" he asked, explaining how she could contaminate the sausage.

"Because I'm not going back to work. I'm going to lunch!"

TODAY: Wash your hands for your own sake, too.

Isn't it amazing how fast dirty jokes spread? And bad news?

Your husband hears a joke in the shop, and, by the time you get to work, everyone on the shift has already heard it!

Likewise, pity the aide who gets called in to the office by the supervisor. Every wing and floor knows her story by the end of the day.

How about spreading joy that fast? Is it possible for good news, for our feelings of happiness and gladness about work, to move quickly through the facility?

The next time you see or hear nice actions or behavior at work, tell others about it. Spread the good word that someone was especially tender to an angry patient, or that a nurse cleaned up a mess instead of asking an aide to do it. Watch what happens. Notice not only how fast news travels, but what it does to everyone's moods and expressions.

TODAY: Bear glad tidings!

When a nursing home or hospital is a truly great place in which to be a patient or an employee, then all the people are satisfied.

Staff do their jobs with pride and a sense of purpose. Patients feel safe and secure. Even visitors to the building can feel the sense of teamwork, the cooperative spirit in the air.

Housekeepers are not just staff who clean the building. They are part of the caregiving team. Few patients know who is a nurses' aide, a kitchen aide, a laundry aide or a housekeeper. Through a patient's eyes, everyone is there to help.

Lynn, a housekeeper for eight years in a 78-patient facility, sighed about how her work is never done. "I clean and clean, and it's still dirty somewhere else." But in the same breath, she added, "But I'm not here just to clean. I'm here because I care about them."

Watching Lynn move about the building with her cart, her care for the patients is obvious. A kind word, a pat on the back, or just stopping to listen to a confused, frail lady, Lynn is part of the caregiving team.

TODAY: See all coworkers as caregivers.

Popular television shows go in cycles. In the early 1960s, westerns were the craze. Then came the spy shows, where handsome men and women lived lives of intrigue. Remember *The Man From Uncle?* Doctor shows, variety shows, lawyer shows. Trends come and go.

In the 1990s, real life dramas of dangerous rescues caught the American public's fancy. Film crews would recapture some horrifying near-tragedy through a reenacted skit, and we would sit spellbound before our televisions.

Cynics would say such a fascination with often bloody, life-threatening events indicates our culture had hit a new low. Theories could be asserted that the average citizen was turned on by pain and suffering, gore and guts.

But what really draws us to these programs is the sheer raw facts—strangers risking their lives to rescue strangers who are at risk of losing their lives. People helping people in the most realistic circumstances.

These daily heroics are the stuff nurses' aides are made of. Minute by minute, twenty-four hours a day, care is lovingly given to strangers, often very fragile strangers.

TODAY: Celebrate your courage.

The well-known anthropologist Desmond Morris was known for his experiments with monkeys. His entertainingly documented research not only revealed a great deal about the lesser primates, it suggested some conclusions about humankind as well.

One such project involved monkeys and art.

Dr. Morris gave a group of monkeys a large canvas and buckets of colorful paint. The monkeys immediately began painting and loved it! They would work for hours without interruption, not even stopping to eat or mate.

To study the monkeys' behavior further, Dr. Morris introduced a reward to the group. Every time they finished a painting, he would give them a treat. Soon, the monkeys stopped making involved, elaborate paintings. Instead, they finished something quickly and waited for their reward. The personal joy of creation they had experienced previously, before they got a reward from someone, was lost.

We're like those monkeys. When we live primarily for the praise and paychecks bestowed by others, we experience little joy or creativity. Rather, we must find our rewards for ourselves and work for the very joy of caring for others.

TODAY: Enjoy inner rewards.

We all need to feel we're making a difference.

As we look back on a tiring day, it is important to recall a few moments when it was clear we helped out. Such a need is at the heart of being a human being— we all need to feel useful, that we are contributing to the greater good.

For patients in nursing homes, while this need has not diminished, the opportunities to serve have been greatly reduced.

No longer working, managing their own homes, paying bills, caring for children or even taking dry clothes off the line, patients can fall into deep depression. Without this sense of value, human beings find little purpose to continue.

Whenever possible, we need to invite our patients to help at whatever level they are able. We can suggest they hold a comb, deliver a message or give us their opinion on something.

On a visit to a large nursing home, I watched a little lady in her wheelchair reach out to a visitor. "Oh, your hands are so cold!" said the patient. "I just came in from outside," the visitor explained. "Would you warm them for me?" The patient beamed, rubbed the stranger's hands vigorously and said, "Anytime! And let me know if I can do anything else for you, okay?"

TODAY: See the caregiver in your patients.

Until the workshop, it didn't seem Elizabeth had ever given her job much thought.

For more than twenty years she had come to work at the same nursing home and had cleaned, bathed, dressed and fed hundreds of patients. She liked the work and hadn't even considered doing anything else. For Elizabeth, life was about being a nurses' aide.

When she was asked what was the greatest part of her work, Elizabeth looked foggy. "The greatest part? What do you mean?" she asked in all honesty, for she had never divided her job into parts. She just liked her job.

Other aides shared their favorite aspects of work, their favorite tasks and/or times. Elizabeth listened.

"I know what I like best!" she smiled, pleased that she had found her answer and eager to share it.

"I like it when my patients are all done up nice!" she said, clasping her hands in her lap and grinning broadly.

TODAY: Notice what makes work special.

In health care, we often read or hear the phrase "the career ladder." Aides can move up to nursing positions, and nurses think about becoming administrators.

Sometimes, employers offer special incentives, so more staff will climb the career ladder. College courses can be paid for, usually after the student passes the class. Often an employee must make a commitment to return to the facility and work for a certain period of time as a kind of payback for the financial assistance.

For some of us, it is the most logical and appropriate step in the world to seek education and earn an LPN or RN degree. Many, many nurses start out as aides.

For others, it is the natural and right decision to stick with our profession and remain a nurses' aide. While others can help us weigh the choices, in the end, each aide must decide alone what is the best move.

One job in health care is not better than another. Even brain surgeons rely on the laundry for totally sterile garb.

Whatever you choose, be proud of what you do.

TODAY: Consider your career in health care.

Ask any furniture maker and they'll tell you that the quality of the wood they work with greatly influences the quality of the tables and chairs they produce.

Aides can relate to this reality.

When getting a patient ready in the morning, it's fun to have a pretty wardrobe to choose from. Selecting a frilly blouse, vibrant plaid shirt or cozy dress can be a nice moment for both the patient and the aide.

Judy didn't enjoy getting one of her patients ready in the morning because the lady's clothes were a disaster.

"They were all worn out, torn, patched, old," said Judy, adding that most of the woman's clothes came from patients who had died.

Judy decided to ask people in a local church if they would like to provide clothes for her patient, not only to donate hand-me-downs, but even to buy a new outfit once in a while. She mentioned this idea to other aides, and before long, a clothing exchange was started.

TODAY: Invite others to share in caring.

March

Pick up any newspaper or news magazine. Someone is getting an award from somebody for doing something. Country musicians, teachers and even folks who have lost a record amount of weight win ribbons and trophies.

Every year the Nobel Prize Committee in Sweden gives out a variety of awards and large cash prizes to individuals from around the world who have excelled in their field. Scientists, poets and playwrights are recognized for their outstanding accomplishments.

Amazingly, half the winners in the science categories share a common achievement—they actually created or invented the category they won! Until they invented the subject, it didn't exist!

Seeing something that others don't see is one of the rare gifts and qualities of being human. The patient Ann thinks is an annoying nuisance is a clever, funny little imp to you. And the man you dread taking care of is Ann's favorite because he reminds her of her grandfather.

By looking at our patients with our own fresh eyes, our own loving ways, our own commitment to our profession, we can discover special characteristics no one else has noticed. We can toast the uniqueness of each person, their precious, one-of-a-kind self.

TODAY: Look for unique qualities in your patients.

In Montpelier the local hardware store is named Somers and Son. The big sign over the front door proclaims that the business is still in the family.

Farmers always pray their sons will follow in their footsteps so the family farm can keep going. And every so often one sees a sign that says "So and so and Daughters."

Such a pattern turns up in nursing homes too. It is not so unusual to find a middle-aged aide with one or more daughters working in the same facility as aides. Choosing the work their mom does is a special tribute to the mom and to the profession.

Aides will often tell stories of how their grandmother or mother took care of elderly relatives at home or in another person's private home. Other aides will share how their brothers, cousins or uncles are firefighters, policemen or some other form of public servant. Coming from a line of caregivers is a proud heritage. Starting such a line, being the first in one's family to provide comfort to those in need, is also a worthy identity.

TODAY: Are you related to other caregivers?

During a panel discussion at a statewide convention of nurses' aides, this question was posed: "What would you do if you walked into a patient's room and he or she was masturbating?"

After the expected nervous laughter and discomfort in the audience, the panel considered the question. "Having noticed what was going on, I would have left the room, closed the door and given him or her their privacy," said Leo, an aide in his thirties.

The audience broke into thunderous applause, pleased that another aide had put patient dignity and rights first.

Sex is a part of life. And nursing homes are places where life very much occurs. People fall in love and sometimes marry, even sharing a room together.

Regardless of why a patient is in a nursing home, we must always remember his or her sense of self and rights have not changed. Patients should not be treated differently or asked to give up any aspect of their self-expression. Rather it is our job to create good conditions for them to have the freedom, privacy and respect all human beings deserve.

TODAY: Respect your patients' sexuality.

Some of us are perfectionists. We conjure up a picture in our mind of what dinner should look like, or how clean the car should stay, or how the conversation in the staff lounge should sound. When things don't go according to our pictures, we get upset.

Taking care of our patients can be the same type of experience. We have a certain image of what a good day looks like. We have a certain pattern we like to follow in putting people to bed.

But somedays, through no fault of our own, things don't work out the way we want.

A coworker goes home to a sick child; a new, withdrawn patient is added to our list; the electricity is knocked out in a storm. Suddenly we lose control and we can't do it all.

"I realize, on those kinds of days, that I can't be all things to all people," said Jane. "And it's hard. I want to do it all, but I can't!"

Being able to see what's happening, that she has to be flexible, is what keeps Jane from losing it. "And if I tell the other girls, they usually pitch in and help me," Jane adds, sharing her other secret to well-being—she doesn't try to do it alone.

TODAY: You're not alone.

A young pastor once told a group of his fellow pastors that he had learned something about human nature that was helping him work with his congregation.

"I read that people generally gain their sense of power or worth in one of three ways—authority, accomplishment or association."

He went on to explain that people who come from a sense of authority often stress their title, their degrees, their visible signs of being in charge.

Those who see their accomplishments as the way they gain their value and attention tend to set goals that will produce satisfaction and success.

The third group, that looks to association as the way to self-worth, needs friendships and relationships to feel okay.

In a nursing home these three groups are well represented. Its easy to look around the building and begin to see who values what. None of the ways are better than another. They simply point out the differences in style between people.

With a little observation, you can begin to figure out which types of people you have trouble with and to which types you are drawn.

TODAY: Recognize and appreciate the differences around you.

Sam was named the state's nursing home volunteer of the year. The competition was tough, but Sam was in a class by himself.

Two and a half years ago Sam had been a patient in the nursing home, having suffered a stroke. The doctors and physical therapists didn't have much hope for Sam.

Incredibly, Sam got stronger. The restraints that had been needed to tie him in the wheelchair were released, and soon he began to walk. After more rehabilitation Sam was told he could return to his wife and home.

But Sam wasn't just a stunning patient; he became a remarkable volunteer. He began volunteering six hours a day, five days a week, working with the staff of the physical therapy unit.

When they nominated him for an award, the patients at the nursing home said weekends were especially hard because they didn't hear Sam's voice.

A retired city policeman, Sam still was drawn to serving others.

TODAY: Hug a volunteer!

Owners of nursing homes insist that they are in the most government-regulated business in the country. While nuclear power may face more rules, nursing homes find that rules, as well as the government funded programs of Medicare and Medicaid, keep them pretty tangled.

The point of this government involvement is protection. The public has demanded that state and federal legislatures pass plenty of laws to insure the safety and well-being of patients.

A patients' bill of rights is part of the law. Education and certification of aides is part of the law. Minimum standards of care are enforced in every home.

Still, these rules can be treated much like a highway speed limit—when no one's looking, how many of us stick to the limit?

The better, higher standard of care that truly guarantees nursing home patients get plenty of good care is one that Donna, an aide for thirty-five years, stated simply, "I take care of them the way I want to be taken care of. And the older I get, the more I really understand what that means."

TODAY: Treat others as you would be treated.

Mary was dying of brain cancer. She was a sweet, pleasant woman who rarely asked for anything.

With her slurred speech it was easy to think Mary had a stroke. One day Mary was asked a routine question by one of her caregivers: "Is there anything I can do for you, Mary?" Surprisingly, Mary answered yes.

She then went on to explain that, the last time her husband had taken her out for a ride, they had gotten a ticket for parking in a handicapped slot without a handicapped plate. Mary felt very badly that her husband, who was just trying to give his wife a little change of scenery, would be fined $25.

The caregiver, while not expecting such a request, said she would see what she could do. She wrote a letter to the mayor, who asked the police to forgive the ticket.

Mary was thrilled.

Often our dying patients need to settle some business to prepare for their own death. We need to be open to their needs, whether they are health-related or not.

TODAY: Listen to your dying patients' need to settle.

In 1987 the federal government passed the most sweeping reform of the nursing home industry in twenty years. Virtually every aspect of the home, from education to room temperature, was addressed.

Probably the most controversial portion of the bill, known as OBRA, called for the release of patients in restraints every two hours, round the clock. Directors of nursing began to calculate what this requirement would mean and quickly figured out the whole day could be consumed in a Chinese fire drill of untying and tying patients.

Several courageous homes decided that the smarter, more humane action would be to simply stop using the restraints entirely. And in fact that is what many began to do.

The benefits to the patients' quality of life were untold. Not only did they have more freedom and independence, but muscle tone improved, as did bladder control.

What started out as an ominous, overwhelming federal mandate became a passport to a better way of life and a more humane nursing practice.

Being broad-minded and willing to try new things can often bring great results.

TODAY: Open your eyes to new approaches.

At the ripe old age of fifty, Ray Kroc founded McDonalds, the most successful chain of restaurants in the world.

Ray, and many other over-fifty entrepreneurs, are good examples for all of us. Other than our own pre-conceptions about age, there is no real reason we can't continue to invent and imagine all of our lives.

Many aides do not enter the work force until they hit their forties or fifties. Raising children, taking care of sick parents or helping a husband with a home business, lots of women don't look outside the home for a challenge until they are alone.

Widowed and/or with grown kids, they begin to look for a place they are needed. Nursing homes are a natural landing strip for these birds flying from their familiar nests. Having cared for loved ones for years, they find the life of a nurses aide a perfect fit. Experienced in how to relax an agitated soul and get a mouth to open wide for dinner, these late bloomers are grand additions to the team.

TODAY: Welcome a new aide!

Every job has its bushel basket of frustrations.

Mechanics might curse nuts they can't pry loose. Librarians dread the long-overdue books.

For nurses' aides the list is varied and vast.

First, the unmentionables. Every family has its code words for the full range of body functions and waste products. Most homes usually develop their own short hand to describe who has done what, which needs to be cleaned up where.

Some aides have more trouble with certain events than with others; usually one or the other end of the anatomy seems worse to them.

Then there are the facility-produced frustrations, such as running out of supplies. It's time to put clean sheets on Mrs. Kollar's bed, and the linen closet is empty! No paper towels in the bathroom either!

At such moments the wise aide just takes a deep breath—maybe five or ten deep breaths! Like a rainy day, some circumstances are beyond our control and rarely worth getting worked up about. Breathe and move on, remembering your purpose.

TODAY: Don't sweat the obvious.

Those who work nights know Albert. Or someone just like him.

Albert begins to stir about 3:30 a.m. And when the clock strikes four there's just no keeping him in bed.

The problem is that the facility does not gear up for the morning routine until six o'clock or even later. So what to do with Albert? Seasoned staff know it is pointless to send him back to bed. He just has to get up.

Some of the new staff can be seen trying to reason with him in the hallway, explaining that the coffee won't be ready until six, that the cook is still at home, that he should be quiet because he is going to wake everybody else.

But Margaret, a nurses' aide all her working life, knows what to do. She goes into the staff lounge, pours a cup of coffee from her own thermos, takes a crumbling muffin out of her bag and goes to Albert.

"Let's sit in here by the window," she tells the old gentleman, his hair tousled from the night. "You can watch the road for cars, watch the people who are leaving early for work. Just like you used to."

Albert smiles proudly. He gets up because he has to, because he always has, because he used to make the donuts. He isn't working at the bakery anymore, but his heart and soul haven't forgotten. He is a working man, a morning man.

Look around you. Chances are those 4 a.m. wanderers are headed out to milk the cows, to drive the bread truck or open the coffee shop.

TODAY: Look for life patterns.

Now one hundred years old, Anna has seen many things in her life taken away. She lost a son in World War II and two husbands to heart attacks. Her vision is nearly gone now, and walking is reserved for trips to the toilet only.

Friends don't call because they are also gone. Dead long ago, their memories are losing their shape and color. Anna has no one to recollect with, because there is no one left with whom she has shared common experiences.

Mail doesn't come. After all, who writes to 100-year-olds? Her 79-year-old nephew is sitting in a dementia unit in another state. He doesn't write letters anymore. What Anna looks forward to is seeing the girls, the women who take care of her. Especially Brenda.

Studying to become an LPN, Brenda likes to study Anna: why she has lived so long, what her secrets are for longevity and good health. Brenda also just plain loves this little wisp of a lady, tucked under the covers like a tiny soft bag of feathers.

Sundays, after she's fed her family, Brenda stops in to visit Anna. After a minute or two of chatter Brenda opens a foil-wrapped baked potato slathered in butter. "I brought you this from home," she says in a hushed voice to Anna.

Anna beams. For reasons she can't understand, baked potatoes have been removed from her diet, and they are her favorite food. And while she has accepted many losses in her life, this one she just couldn't take. Thanks to Brenda, she doesn't have to.

 TODAY: Consider your patient's losses.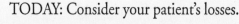

In Montana a program called Chalice of Repose brings special music to the bedside of dying patients.

The concept is simple, having been adapted from the first hospices established in European monasteries for dying monks. The soothing, beautiful chants and harp solos filled the monastery rooms with peace and harmony. Comfort and artistic expression replaced pain and fear.

Chalice of Repose volunteers today refer to their work as "death midwifery"—they are ushering the terminally ill into their next life or place. Though death is a personal and singular event, not unlike birth, others can make the moment less frightening and more comfortable.

Healthcare workers, when assigned to the deathbeds of frail patients, are midwives too. Yes, dying is something every person does alone, but the attention and care brought into the room can transform the final days from times of loneliness and fear to sweet moments of loving ministration.

Voices become musical instruments, cooing softly as chores are done for the patient. The calming hum of conversation sings like a harp, relaxing the troubled patient, allowing him or her to peacefully let go of this world.

Serving a dying man or woman is a rare and precious honor. Being part of such an intimate scene permits us to love powerfully and unconditionally, assuring our patients that all is right with this world and it is all right to go on to the next.

TODAY: See the privilege of your work.

Human beings need changes in scenery.

Young mothers know this fact well, often having learned it the hard way. How to keep the baby from crying? Push that stroller! Spin that mobile! Find something else in your purse to amuse him!

Variety of scenery is generally unavailable to those confined in hospitals and nursing homes. Even the homebound elderly or "shut-ins" know this truth—it gets pretty boring. Television sets and windows become necessities.

For the staff, scenery remains varied and stimulating since, every day, you get to leave and experience the world beyond the building walls. No matter how routine and repetitive the work or the surroundings, come 7 a.m., 3 p.m., 11 p.m., or whatever time the shift ends, freedom and visual variety return.

Imagine what you would feel like if today, at the precise time you are putting on your coat and heading for the door, somebody yells, "Hey, where do you think you're going? Get back in here. And get back in your room."

Imagine this new predicament—that this is to be your home, but that you will not be permitted to go back out there, into your car, on the road, into the mall. Imagine that you must limit yourself to the scenery you are all too familiar with, that this is it.

No wonder patients get agitated, irritable, depressed.

TODAY: Forgive cabin fever.

March 16

In his book *In Wisdom and Grace,* Raymond Stovich talks about working with Hilda, a chronic wanderer who exasperated her family and healthcaregivers.

Her trips on foot were accompanied by her stories, stories she told over and over again. She didn't seem to tire of her stories or of her need to wander.

Working with Dr. Stovich, Hilda developed a small model of the area in the town where she wanted to wander. They built a series of familiar buildings and streets and got a small plastic figure to be Hilda.

Hilda then was encouraged to walk her small "self" through the diorama and to tell the stories as she did so. As she passed the dress shop, she talked of her first prom dress. The five-and-dime had a soda bar inside where she took her children and grandchildren in the summer. The jewelry store was where Hilda's late husband presented her engagement ring.

Dr. Stovitch writes that Hilda was at first hesitant about walking through this tiny town and telling her tales. Then she began to reminisce. Some of the stories changed with the telling, as if she was working out some aspect of her past.

A granddaughter taped one of these memory sessions, and other family members became interested in developing their family history. Hilda joined an exercise group to use some of the energy that used to be devoted to wandering. "Within a few weeks Hilda's wandering had disappeared, replaced by a sophisticated act of the imagination, and her personal feelings of well-being and happiness were at an all time high."

TODAY: Listen in a new way.

St. Patrick's Day!

As many an Irish uncle has been heard to say, any excuse for a party.

If your employer permits street clothes on the job, today is a fun day to study your closet and drawers for all green clothes. No outfit is too absurd; your patients and coworkers will love it!

For those who wear uniforms the challenge is a bit greater. But don't be discouraged. I still remember Danny, who dyed his hair green for our total pleasure. Green earrings, socks, shoes, nail polish, and other accessories can make you a proud Irishman too.

Or better yet, get an inexpensive bottle of foundation make-up. (Remember, we used to call it pancake make-up? There is probably an old bottle in your medicine cabinet!)

Get to work fifteen minutes early today. Bring the make-up and some green food coloring to work, along with a small watercolor brush or make-up brush.

Set up a decorating station. Mix some foundation in a paper cup with a few drops of coloring. And let the games begin! A shamrock on the cheek is always successful! And spotted leprechaun rash is quite contagious. Patients and staff have been known to catch it quite quickly.

TODAY: Get green!

V. Beverly Nickles, a gerontologist and staff trainer from Georgia, has done some fascinating research with nurses' aides in the southern United States.

As part of her master's degree at Appalachian State University, Ms. Nickles surveyed nurses' aides in several states about why they left their work. It seems that, nationwide, the turnover in this profession still remains close to 100 percent! Maybe you won't leave your job, but another position in the facility is filled three times in the year, hence the averages.

To everyone's surprise the Nickles study revealed an unexpected piece of information. Aides who were leaving the job identified the number one reason for quitting as an inability to deal with death.

Labeled "death anxiety" in the literature, this syndrome makes it harder and harder to handle patients' deaths. Feeling sad, angry and helpless, the aide seeks another, less painful job.

Actually, to feel badly about death is normal! It means we really love the patient. The trick here is to also see the inevitable event as normal. Rather than regard death as the enemy, a sign of a caregiver's failure, the challenge is to realize this life-step is out of our hands. We simply must love our patients, and, when they are gone, continue to love their memory.

TODAY: Remember, death is a condition of life.

During a moment of almost stinging honesty, a young aide named Molly confessed to other staff that she had been making fun of one of the laundry workers.

"Her last name is Leo, and we call her B.O.," she said awkwardly, explaining how badly Ms. Leo smelled. The rest of the staff tittered a bit nervously. This was not news. They too had used that nickname, and a few others too.

One sure sign of our humanness is gossip. We hate it and we love it. We hate it when it is about us or we are caught. We may even hate it just because we know it is cruel. But we love it when it is funny or secretive. After all, it is no accident that the *National Enquirer* and *People Magazine* sell out every week. We love gossip!

But behind this love is really a simple longing to be close to others, to know one another and be near. Perhaps, instead of telling her coworkers about Ms. Leo/B.O., Molly can go to her and say, "Pat, this is really hard for me, but I want to talk with you privately for a minute. I want you to know that people are talking about your body odor, and if they were talking about me, I would want to know."

Kindness of this sort will bring the best kind of closeness into Molly's life—friendship built on honesty and caring.

Spread no gossip. When someone offers it, ask "Why are you telling me?"

TODAY: Derail the gossip train.

Anyone who thinks being a nurses' aide is about making sure patients are dry, warm and fed is right.

Now the rest of the story!

Providing your patients with the basics is like doing the same things for yourself—your day is about a lot more than eating, sleeping and using the bathroom.

What you are really called to do, what your work is truly about, doesn't even appear on your job description. How could they write "love creatively"? But, done well, that is what your work is about.

Old Martha was an odd old bird. She had phantom friends she talked to all day, rambling in and out of lengthy conversations. She was always jabbering. Alert patients avoided her. Her few visitors felt uncomfortable, would stay a few minutes and leave. Everyone wanted to do something for Martha, but she seemed unreachable, locked inside her own mind.

Until Kim came to work. A new nurses' aide, she wasn't fully sure what she was supposed to do for patients. It seemed there was plenty to do and always a little more on top of that.

But one day she brought an old telephone from home and taped the cord to the wall of Martha's room.

"Your friend Katherine is on the phone for you," Kim told old confused Martha.

Martha's face cleared like a TV screen with a new antenna.

"Why thank you!" she exclaimed, taking the phone.

After a long conversation—Martha spoke both parts—she hung up contentedly. And sat silently.

Silently! From that day forward Martha would choose to use her phone when she needed to talk. She called old friends from far and wide and talked over all of her memories. Her jabbering ended.

TODAY: Love creatively.

During orientation Alice was introduced to some of the patients. Alice had worked as an aide in Connecticut and had just moved to Vermont. This was her first day in the small facility.

"This is Betty," Alice was told.

Betty was dressed in a pink, stained, sweat-suit and tennis shoes. She had no teeth. Her short hair was matted. She was bone-thin, bent and seemed intent on walking somewhere. When someone said her name, Betty didn't react. She spent her time reacting to things going on inside herself. As Alice watched Betty travel through the home, she began to wonder how she could relate to this far away lady.

The facility orientation continued.

"Betty was a lawyer in the Sacco-Vanzetti trial. Do you know about that?"

Alice said no. The trainer then shared the story of this fascinating case which ended with death sentences for two alleged murderers.

For Alice, Betty's intensity and deliberate walk now made sense. No, she would probably never hear first hand of the trial or any other part of Betty's life. But she could hold this image and experience in her mind and could use it to remind herself when she was caring for Betty.

TODAY: Respect your patient's lives.

Part of public school education usually includes field trips to places in the community such as fire stations and hospitals. Our children are also sometimes asked to have their parents come to school and talk about what they do for a living.

The next time you can, why not get a group of aides together and offer to speak to a class?

Kids need to hear about your important work. They need to understand what happens when we get old in America. They need to begin considering this work as something they might like to do.

Invite your son's or daughter's (or grandchild's!) class to tour your facility. If you are too shy to lead the tour, talk to your director of nursing or your activities director about hosting the class. Perhaps they could help with a program like bingo or painting?

Yours is a proud profession of selfless individuals who work long, tough hours for less than enough pay. The society doesn't reward you enough for your labors, but that shouldn't stop you from feeling good about who you are and what you do. Without you, the folks living in institutions across this country wouldn't exist. They would be props, bags tied to chairs, waiting.

As the population of the elderly continues to grow, we will need more caregivers than ever before. Become a recruiter!

TODAY: Educate your children proudly.

Studies show almost 60 percent of a nurse's time is spent doing paperwork. As government regulations become more and more demanding, the nurse must devote more and more of each day to paper compliance, making sure that complete records are kept on everything that happens in the home.

It is not unusual to see, hanging in a shower room, charts detailing patients' bowel movements! Nothing goes undocumented.

Given the amount of time nurses are anchored at the desk, the aide's job becomes all the more critical. After all, the aide is not only the primary caregiver; the aide is the eyes of the nursing staff.

If a patient seems funny, different from the usual, tell the nurses. Go with your gut. Some nurses may act as if you are a darn nuisance, as if you are stepping out of bounds.

You need to trust your judgment. So what if sometimes you are told to back off or mind your own business? Another time you just might be the reason a patient is diagnosed as having had a stroke during the night.

Tune yourself to your patients. Variations in their normal routines can mean something is happening with them. If the patient who always wants to be first out of bed and dressed before 9 o'clock is refusing to rise, pay attention. Your work includes such observation.

TODAY: Pay attention to changes.

At an informal gathering of caregivers, someone asked, "What are the three most important things you need to know in your work?"

After some thought, a man who had been running a board and care home for twenty years with his wife said: patience, patience, patience. He elaborated that this amount of patience was needed for dealing with his residents, their families and the government. Everyone had advice for him and most had complaints too. He needed to remain patient to be able to work with all of the parties involved.

Across the table, a nurse who had also worked twenty years said, "I agree with John. But I spell my answer `patients, patients, patients.'"

She went on to explain that, for her, the key to a meaningful career had been to get to know all her patients fully. She always becomes familiar with them, their lives, their families, their health. Equipped with this knowledge, she feels she can best serve them.

Healthcare is a demanding field. Unlike the plumber or computer operator, you work with objects that talk back and have feelings. What are the three things you think are most important to your work?

TODAY: Be patient with your patients.

Ray had been a vegetable farmer all his life. He supervised crews that worked on hundreds of acres of plants, growing all kinds of beans, squash, potatoes. He rotated his crops and fed plenty of people.

As a farmer, Ray's life was about being outdoors. He was a man who studied the skies, who wanted to talk about the weather, the changing seasons, the climate. But now Ray was living in a nursing home in the city. He no longer rode a tractor; a wheelchair was his transportation.

Cooking for 150 patients, the kitchen used huge cans of canned vegetables. The only fresh vegetables Ray seemed to get, tomatoes, tasted like hard rubber balls to him. Sam was Ray's main aide. He was also a gardener. One night, while planting his own tomatoes after work, Sam had an idea.

The next morning Sam arrived at Ray's room with a packet of seeds, a bag of potting soil and an old dishpan. "Ray," Sam said. "It's time to plant the tomatoes!"

Very little else was said. Ray put his hands into the dirt, holding it like the hand of a lost friend. He knew what to do.

Over the weeks and months, the tomato plants developed a large and devoted audience. Few folks could visit the home without checking on Ray's Babies. And when the day came for harvest, the kitchen managed to get some very fresh lettuce from the farmers' market, and Ray enjoyed an old favorite, a toasted BLT. So did Sam.

TODAY: Sow and reap.

Yikes! This is the day that strikes fear into the hearts of all staff! The state inspectors are here.

Generally registered nurses, these inspectors or surveyors are trained to evaluate the care delivered in your facility. They are thorough in their review, studying every aspect of the day to day operation. How are the onions stored? What temperature is the hot water? Have aides received training in patient rights? Do the patients feel their rights are respected?

In homes where quality has slipped below the acceptable minimums, the inspectors ask for specific improvements. Written reports are made, and plans of correction must be designed and completed.

Working for the state, and sometimes for the federal government, the inspectors are responsible for assuring their employers that care in nursing homes is good. Technically, while you and the inspectors work for different organizations, you are both responsible for the same thing—good patient care.

In fact, because most people who live in nursing homes are unable to pay for their care, tax dollars are used to pay their way and your salaries. Tax dollars are used to pay for the inspectors too.

Thus you not only share a common commitment to quality and a common concern for patients, you share the same boss—the taxpayer.

TODAY: See commonalities.

An owner of a small nursing home first pointed out the phenomenon to me.

"Did you ever notice that quiet people tend to work nights?" Ted asked.

In his more than forty years in long term care work, he had developed this theory. He watched people come and go, ask for changes in assignments, settle into their comfortable routine as employees. As important as the right job and the right coworkers, in Ted's mind, is the right shift.

Are you someone who enjoys quiet? Do you look forward to that time just before the sun goes down, that dusky evening sky when everything seems to slow down and get still?

Or is the ritual of the morning your favorite time? Are you the first one up, making the coffee and preparing the house for another day? Do you like to walk the dog at dawn?

Knowing something about your own innate personality can be most useful when looking for your niche in the nursing home. If you're "not a morning person," why put yourself, your colleagues and most importantly, the residents, through a rotten morning with sleepy you? Show up at 7 p.m., you night owl!

TODAY: Notice your needs.

To the visitor, Harold was a most pleasant man, almost gracious. He frequently sat by the main entrance, greeting people as they entered or exited. Not a highly talkative man, Harold was simply polite.

When the aides reported Harold to be a difficult patient, it was hard to believe.

"He hits and swears; I'm afraid of him at bath time," said Sandy. The other aides agreed, joking they would do about anything to get out of bathing Harold.

"Harold? Sweet Harold?" the wide-eyed consultant asked, gesturing to the kindly gentleman stationed in the foyer.

"Yup," the staff maintained.

Sitting alone, the consultant asked Harold to tell her about his life. Where had he worked? Where had he lived?

Harold had been an office worker all his life, sitting at a desk eight hours a day. His family life? "Why I never married. Neither did my brother. We lived together until he died two years ago."

After a few more statements it became clear— Harold had no experience living with women, let alone being bathed by them!

A few changes in the staff schedule were made, and the kindly old gentleman was assigned a male aide at bath time. At ease with his caregiver, Harold had no reason to act out.

TODAY: Watch for cues and clues.

Reduced to living in one room, often with a stranger, nursing home residents can keep very few personal possessions with them.

One most prized item always moves in with them, though, and that is their name.

So many of the names are incredible and one-of-a-kind: Losetta, Saba, Granthia, Tump.

Caught up in your own thoughts and list of things to do, it's pretty easy to go through the motions of caregiving and just plain forget to be with your patient.

Asking about the meaning of someone's name, or how they got their name, can lead to some wonderful, personal conversations.

Sometimes we learn about a name that has been in a family for generations, or how their mother and dad invented the name by merging their own. Sometimes we learn it is a nickname, given by a baby brother or sister who just couldn't say "Kingsley" so they said "Kip."

Being interested in someone is a very high compliment. Listening to their stories can be a treasured time. And you just may learn something too.

TODAY: Ask about an unusual name.

As the gardener at Pine Manor, Fred didn't spend much time with patients; he had said more than once that he would talk to a plant before he would talk to a patient. Fred's attitude was not that uncommon. Maintenance, laundry, dietary and even office staff often tended to be separate. Their mind-set was, "Nurses and aides work with the patients; we don't."

Everything changed when Mr. Grout came to live at Pine Manor. His family had cared for him as long as they could at their home, but now, in the advanced stages of Alzheimer's, Mr. Grout needed twenty-four-hour supervision. There was no telling where he would go or what he would be found doing. Given Mr. Grout's ability to cruise over great distances in a short period of time and his severe dementia, the director of nursing at Pine Manor wrote a special care plan.

"The entire staff must be a part of Mr. Grout's care," she wrote. "All employees will look after his well-being."

Fred the gardener quickly became a caregiver one cold November morning. Salting the icy walk, he watched Mr. Grout walk into the front yard, drop his pants, and begin to relieve himself on a pile of leaves. Alerting the staff by walkie-talkie, Fred was told, "We need your help Fred. Go ahead and help him into the house."

At first resistant, over time Fred saw he actually enjoyed his work more, now that he knew some patients by name. Later he even learned the care of roses from one of the patients.

TODAY: Treat all employees as team players.

Reporting a fellow worker for drinking on the job is not easy. It is, however, essential.

Marilyn had suspected her friend Lois of bringing booze to work. Some days she thought she could smell something on Lois's breath. "Maybe it's just from last night," Marilyn hoped.

One Tuesday morning Marilyn couldn't ignore her suspicions any longer. Getting a patient ready for her shower, Lois had nearly dropped the little woman. Lois seemed confused and unable to keep her balance. Marilyn helped Lois finish the patient's care and then pulled her into the staff bathroom.

"Lois, I believe you have been drinking," Marilyn said, adding that she was worried for everyone's sake. "I want you to go talk to the head nurse, or I will have to for you."

Angry and defensive, Lois lashed out at Marilyn, calling her names and denying her charges. "I'm on cold medicine," Lois claimed.

Thinking over the incident, Marilyn recalled the rules of the job and the commitment she had made when hired. "Report all patient abuse, even if you only suspect it." This was potential abuse, and Marilyn reported it.

TODAY: Protect your patients, not abusive staff.

April

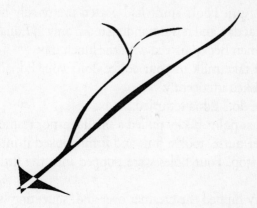

April 1

"Today at exactly 12 noon I will milk a cow in Edna's room!" announced Becky, an aide who always had a joke for her patients.

"Sounds good to me, " said Edna, a farm girl who loved talk of barns and cows and hot chocolate made with thick unpasteurized milk.

The April Fool's spirit had gotten pretty silly by noon that day, and it was standing room only in Edna's room when Becky arrived with the lunch tray.

"You take milk in your coffee don't you, Edna?" Becky asked innocently.

"Sure do," Edna returned.

At that point Becky pulled a small plastic creamer from her purse, took a fork and firmly poked it into the foil top. Four holes were popped into the little serving.

Becky flipped the creamer over and, squeezing its sides, shot four streams of milk into Edna's cup. "There, I milked it!" she laughed.

TODAY: Do something silly and fun.

Let's face it, we all love to eat. Just watch television for one night and see how many advertisements push delicious, scrumptious food—hamburgers, pizzas, ice cream, cookies, soda. The list is as long as the grocery aisles.

Most of us are on diets some part of the year. Even if we aren't eating food, we are thinking about it. Graduations, weddings, Halloween, birthdays, and even church, include coffee and goodies. Our kids grow up with three meals a day and snacks too. And almost as a tradition they all complain about school lunches.

Is it any wonder that meals are big deals in nursing homes?

Given the limited number of things that happen in an average nursing home to an average patient on an average day, mealtime can take on an even greater role. No matter how flat the day, patients know that at least three times they will be greeted with an unknown and potentially pleasant experience.

Not unlike the rest of America, patients find eating means real excitement. Mealtime is a social time.

As staff, it is important we not rush people, forcing them to gobble food at breakneck speeds. When possible, alert residents who enjoy conversation should be seated together. Appropriate seating should be created for folks who get pretty messy, so they have privacy and no one's appetite is upset!

Making meals pleasant benefits everyone. Not only do we feed our patient's physical needs, we care for their general well-being as well.

 TODAY: Enjoy meal time.

Traditionally nursing has been a female profession. Nationally, only three percent of the registered and licensed nurses are men. The statistics for nurses' aides are believed to be about the same.

Caregiving, like teaching, has historically been a field regarded as acceptable employment for women. Considered by some as extensions of mothering, these two fields are still dominated by women.

However, with the expansion of the women's movement in the 1970s, the career world for women began to expand. Today women continue to enter workplaces previously labeled "all male." These changes mean fewer women are choosing healthcare, causing some employers to worry about a shortage of good workers.

Men who join a predominantly female staff, often taking care of predominantly female patients, are unusual individuals. They are willing to face society's sometimes demeaning view of male caregivers. They also must face the staff lounge dynamics of being greatly outnumbered.

Yet, knowing these obstacles, they still choose caregiving because they also know of the great rewards.

TODAY: Acknowledge male staff.

Doc was in his nineties and withdrawing more and more from the reality around him. He seemed to sit for hours in his comfortable chair gazing somewhere inside. When greeted, he would jump, as if stirred from deep concentration.

Holding a doctorate in music, not medicine, Doc was a lifelong cellist. Only one staff member, however, had heard Doc play, as that little performance occurred long ago when different people worked at the home.

Introducing Doc to a visitor, a compassionate staff member named Sally suggested they open the case and look at the cello. His beautiful French style instrument lay in the well-worn case. The broken and loose hairs of the bow stuck out wildly.

"This bow needs to be rehaired!" the visitor said, and Doc, while still somewhat foggy, seemed to understand and agree. "I must take it tonight to...," Doc said, his voice trailing off with the thought.

Later, Sally arranged for the bow to be rehaired, and, a few weeks later, it was back in Doc's hands. He didn't choose to play that day, but he was clearly pleased with the whole situation. Rocking slightly from side to side, clapping the tips of his fingers together, Doc watched everything. "You're pretty excited, aren't you Doc?" Sally asked with a loving smile. Several evenings later, some short, disconnected strains of cello music could be heard from a room on the third floor. Doc was reconnecting with a part of himself and his life that had been forgotten.

TODAY: Help a patient find a lost love.

Edna Wilder wrote a wonderful book about her mother: *Once upon an Eskimo Time: A Year of Eskimo Life Before the White Man Came As Told To Me By My Wonderful Mother Whose Eskimo Name was Nedercook.*

Nedercook, known in Alberta, Canada, as Grandma Tucker, lived to the remarkable age of one-hundred and twenty-one years. Growing up on the Bering Strait in a truly primitive culture, her life story is amazing. Her life included no conveniences; they ate what they killed. The book describes Nedercook's tenth year and is filled with the hunting expeditions, the rituals, and the songs of her childhood.

As an adult, Grandma Tucker was equally fascinating. At age 108 she broke her hip and was told by doctors that she would never walk again.

Grandma Tucker could not accept this, of course, but was too embarrassed to use the walker in the hospital while others were watching. She waited until everyone else had gone to bed and then walked up and down the corridors alone, practicing until she was well enough to trade in the walker for a cane, then giving that up eventually.

Do we make our patients too embarrassed to try? Do we take away their hope by our expressions or attitudes? Do we tell them they will never do something again?

TODAY: Believe in your patients.

Depending on who you ask and how honest they feel, the percentage of depressed people living in nursing homes runs from "some" to "most."

And why wouldn't they be? We live in a culture that says you are your work and your health. If you're not working or not well, you aren't important. Just think back to those times you were unemployed or sick. You felt rotten, like half a person. Your patients struggle every day with this same loss of their identities. Without a job and good health they feel like they don't exist.

Professor James Sykes of the University of Wisconsin Medical School, speaking before the World Federation for Mental Health (August 1991), shared his research on the subject of patient depression.

His research led him to conclude that, to help improve the mental well-being of older persons, caregivers must help their patients "put their work and their health in perspective. They are neither their work, nor their health—whether stated in positive terms or negatives losses." Dr. Sykes stresses the need to focus on the life values that last a lifetime, not just those tied to our prime time years.

Beyond emphasizing the lasting values, Dr. Sykes suggests caregivers help older people cope with their losses by inviting them to tell their stories.

As they do, they seem to develop greater personal strength and increase their self-esteem. This finding, indicated by hundreds of intensive conversations with older people, confirms the results of this most recent investigation. As our elders tell their stories they explore what may be described as their spiritual journey.

TODAY: Invite stories.

According to the Lyceum graduates at the Holiday House in St. Albans, one is never too old to learn.

A curious bunch of women, average age ninety, these nursing home patients decided there were some subjects they wanted to know more about, such as prisoners of war and Judaism. Their energetic activities director, Alice Astleford, assembled a faculty for the course, which totaled thirty hours of class time. Retired military men, rabbis, teachers and business leaders gladly donated their time and expertise, tutoring the eager students about the subjects they had chosen.

Upon completing the course (there were no dropouts!) the students planned a grand commencement. Held in the evening in the large function room, the event attracted families, staff and even the local press. The National Honor Society provided ushers for each graduate, the high school music director handled the music, and the facility ordered corsages for all graduates. Most striking were the purple caps and gowns sold (at cost) for $5 each by the owner of the gown company (who said he had never heard of such a neat ceremony).

I was thrilled to be the commencement speaker, though I felt I had little I could tell these wise women other than to praise the fact that they made aging look fun.

The class will was read, with each graduate giving her wishes for the others in the facility. It was a glorious evening, topped off with a front page picture in the morning paper.

TODAY: Encourage learning!

In the days of hippies and love beads, schools attempted to adapt their teaching styles. Students were offered sensitivity training and "T" (therapy) groups in which to express their true feelings.

Warm fuzzies and cold pricklies became code words for kind and cruel words and deeds.

Whatever we think of these methods today, some aspects made a lot of sense. Everyone needs to be able to express what is going on within themselves. And we all would prefer kind to cruel words.

Talk with other aides about creating some symbolic warm fuzzies for the facility. What could you exchange? A church camp uses little cotton balls. Everyone gets a few at the beginning of camp, to be given freely to whomever they think needs to have a little treat to feel good about themselves.

A little jar of your "currency" could sit next to the time card machine. Grab a few cotton balls or paper hearts and give them to both staff and residents when they look like they need a lift.

TODAY: Give some warm fuzzies.

Statistics tabulated by the US Department of Labor consistently reveal a disturbing fact—nursing homes report the third largest number of occupational injuries and illnesses.

The only other workplaces with a greater level of claims are the meat processing factories and motor vehicle plants. Interestingly enough, these other high reporting industries are manufacturing concerns.

Why is your work such a high-risk field? Do staff subconsciously suffer injuries so they can take a paid break from the exhausting demands of the work? Do we, again in our subconscious, seek to leave the job but feel too guilty to quit?

The common explanations for the high workers' compensation claims in this industry generally center on heavy lifting and untrained staff. If that's the case, it seems the statistics could be lowered consistently through education. If, however, the reasons for lost work time and injury are more subtle and hidden, reducing this industry's standing will take some work on the part of a lot of individuals. Watch your work habits and routines. When do accidents happen? Why? When do you get sick? Following or preceding what? Begin to hear what your body is telling you.

TODAY: Listen to your body's needs.

No one could understand why Eunice was freaking out. This quiet, almost shy lady had lived in the home for nearly five years. Other than a few yelling incidents when she was in pain with a urinary tract infection, she had never been labeled a behavior problem.

But today Eunice had that label—written in big, red letters. Ever since she had been moved to another wing, she had been agitated, acting out and striking staff. The mystery seemed to be tied to the move from A wing to B wing.

The administrator had made sure the caregivers remained the same and that her roommate would move with her. All of the rooms in the facility were the same size and design.

In reviewing Eunice's past, her interests and hobbies, an aide stumbled on a clue—Eunice had once been an avid gardener. Even in her first few years at the home, she had spent a little time in the yard tending to the small rose garden.

That was it! Looking out the window of her old room, Eunice could see the garden. The sight of this familiar scene gave her great comfort and a solid sense of well-being. Without that view she felt disoriented and alone.

TODAY: Notice the little things.

Depending on the economy and what part of the country you live in, nurses and aides may be in great demand. During those times of low unemployment, facilities may turn to nursing agencies or rental pools. Operating on the Kelly Girl principle, pools provide nursing homes with temporary staff.

For the residents and permanent staff, the inclusion of strangers in the work routine can be disruptive and even unsettling.

Rental aides can be paid almost twice what permanent staff receive, as the substitutes get no benefits. This inequity can cause hard feelings and resentment.

Further, a resident being bathed by a stranger can become very ill at ease. Bath time is always tough, but adding the dynamic of a stranger unfamiliar with personal preferences and needs compounds the difficulties.

The temptation for facility staff, of course, is not to cooperate with the agency employee. Human nature makes it pretty natural to hope the substitute falls on her face.

Such an unwelcoming response, while understandable, is obviously damaging. Patient care is jeopardized when we don't work as a team. The role of permanent staff is not to thwart the subs, or put them in the wrong. The point is to create a sense of team and to work for the common good, the care of frail residents.

TODAY: Build team with all staff.

Growing attached to certain patients is natural and unavoidable. Management can tell you all they want that having favorites is not allowed. You know what your heart tells you!

When one of our pet patients is dying, we sometimes feel we can't take the job another day. Seeing someone we love go downhill is painful. Especially when we like to make people comfortable and meet their needs. Not being able to make things all better, to bring about a happy ending, is a bitter reality.

Bethany Bell, an aide at Rowan Court Nursing Home, struggled with this feeling of helplessness. The patient she was closest to was dying and Bethany felt powerless. What could she do?

Working with the administrator, Bethany designed TLC, a voluntary program that aides can join. If an aide would like to sit at the death bed of a particular patient, he or she merely signs up for a paid eight-hour shift. Rowan Court staff report they have much less anxiety about death, perhaps because they have a choice.

Not being able to be with a loved one, to say goodbye, leaves one feeling incomplete. The phenomenon is sometimes referred to as "not being able to bury your dead." Family will tell you this is why a funeral service helps.

Being aware of our own feelings and needs during a time of death can make the sadness bearable.

TODAY: Design solutions.

If you looked closely you could see the gleaming spot on Margaret's shoulder was a tiny gold angel.

A cheerful woman who had raised a large family, Margaret was full of joy. Her broad smile was genuine and dependable. When Margaret came to work, she came with her smile.

Working alongside this happy lady, one couldn't help but wonder what her secret might be. A few coworkers cynically wrote Margaret off as a kook; one even called her a "Jesus Freak."

The patients never considered her a kook, though. Margaret was a kind, cool breeze that blew in and out of their room, bringing comfort and good tidings. She was missed on her days off and welcomed home when she returned.

"What is your secret, Margaret?" a new aide asked. "How do you stay up?"

Amused by the sense of the supernatural surrounding the query, Margaret laughed softly. "No secret, dear," she said straightforwardly. "I let my hands lead with love. And when they need a lift, I remember I have an angel on my shoulder, and she takes over."

TODAY: Put an angel on your shoulder.

Like baseball teams, nursing homes are only as good as their staff.

State inspectors come and go, training programs begin and end, supervisors go on and off the floor. Much of the time, staff are on their own, whizzing through the halls, checking tasks off their list.

Unfortunately, some of us are unable to work at a high level of performance when left alone. Our nature calls us to slow down, to take the easy way out, even to cut corners.

In one Connecticut River facility, nurses' aides were putting patients to bed with their shoes on! Why? "To make getting them up in the morning easier!"

Incredible as this logic seems, at least five employees thought this procedure made sense. Driven by the tremendous work load and the sense that "you're behind before you start," these aides were desperately looking for some relief from the pace.

While such treatment can not be condoned, it can be understood. Facilities need to tune in to these kinds of mistakes, for they symbolize something larger. The issue is greater than shoes worn to bed; the issue involves the staff members' inner ability to make wise judgments. Also involved here is the need to give staff a reasonable workload which they can handle and feel good about.

TODAY: Make wise judgments.

Income taxes are due and Ben Franklin's wisdom rings out: "The only things certain are death and taxes."

In the nursing home, about 20 percent of our patients do go home, but we can be pretty certain that most will die in our care. Our residents know this, and perhaps this fact is precisely why folks resist being admitted to a nursing home. They know it is most likely their last home.

Communities have carved out interesting locations for nursing homes. Usually you can find one near the hospital—and don't be surprised if there is a cemetery around the corner. The dynamics are striking. Looking out one's hospital window, it is possible to see one's final home and one's final resting place.

At the Vermont Veterans' Home the cemetery is in the front yard. There the fallen soldiers lie, buried by mourning family and friends.

The presence of this burial ground is a constant reminder to patients of their mortality, of the finite nature of their stay. For staff the tombstones out the window serve another purpose as reminders of the brevity of life. As death is a condition of life, the nursing home staff must strive to make each day a full day. Caring for frail people, we must seek to make each day enough, complete, able to stand on its own. Our patients must feel loved, safe and secure. And whatever life they have in them must be lived.

TODAY: Let death make life precious.

In planning a joint project with nurses' aides, a group of nurses began talking about the value of nurses' aides establishing an association. Continuing education, determining standards, feeling good about their work and attracting others to the career were listed as potential benefits of such an organization.

"I want my aides to go to the nurse aide association meetings because they will be encouraged to be more professional," said Maggie, a director of nursing.

"Nurses' aides aren't professionals. Their work is not a profession," another director countered.

Defined as "a body of persons engaged in an occupation or calling," the word profession connotes a group of people committed to a common mission. If that isn't an aide, what is?

Most of the care in a nursing home is delivered by aides. These employees are required by federal law to complete seventy-five hours of training. In some states, more than a hundred hours are required. Upon successfully passing the standardized test, the aide is deemed a certified nurses' aide.

Many aides have made this vocation their life's work—twenty, thirty, even forty years' worth. To consider aides anything other than professionals is demeaning and unacceptable. It also smacks of paternalism and a caste system.

For years nurses have regarded doctors as looking down on them. Do nurses also feel they should look down on aides? The fact is that the best places to live and work are homes where everyone respects everyone else, where all employees are regarded as competent professionals.

TODAY: Celebrate your profession.

The volunteer banquet at Linden Lodge is always a spectacular event. A special evening set aside to toast those citizens who give time and talent to the nursing home, the banquet brings some real characters together.

This year a mother-daughter team of belly dancers joined the crowd of celebrants.

In her sixties, Kay, the mom, laughed about how she got into belly dancing. "Well, my daughter has done it for years, and she kept telling me I would like it. So I tried it and I love it!"

Apparently the patients really love her too.

"Whenever we go to dance, the patients tell me that they like me best!" said Kay. "They won't stand for it if I don't perform!"

Seeing Kay's impish grin and mischievous eyes, it's not hard to figure out her appeal. This playful lady is about having fun, enjoying, partying. No matter where we live, we all love a party. Kay's slinky colorful outfit and pixie personality make her the people's choice. As my grandmother always said, "If you want to be happy, be around happy people!"

TODAY: Invite an entertainer to the facility.

Old Winnie the Pooh and Piglet have a lot to teach us.

Not thought of as literature for those who work with the elderly, nevertheless these two creatures have a message for all caregivers.

In A.A. Milne's *The House at Pooh Corner*, Pooh and Piglet are taking a walk through the Hundred Acre Woods.

"Pooh," whispers Piglet.

"Yes," answers Pooh. "What is it?"

"Oh nothing," says Piglet, taking Pooh's paw. "I just wanted to be sure of you."

In that brief exchange, A.A. Milne's animals speak for all of us who are walking along life's path, this Hundred Acre Wood. We don't want to think we are alone. We want to feel safe and secure, that someone is there if and when we need them, that we are not alone.

When our patients reach out for us, for a reassuring word or touch, we need to be sensitive to the little Piglet in all of us. The part of our self which worries we aren't likable or, worse yet, aren't lovable.

TODAY: Let your patients be sure of you.

Wesley healthcare Center in Saratoga Springs, NY, has written what they label "a statement of culture." In it the facility tries to answer the question, "What makes Wesley healthcare Center?"

The two page document speaks to physical and spiritual well-being, death with dignity and the individual's right to make decisions about his or her life.

Attempting to quantify or write down a home's identity is a brave undertaking. What does the home stand for? What is its position in the community and in the lives of the people who live and work there?

For you as an employee, nearly half of your waking hours are spent in this place. What have you associated yourself with? What are you furthering? What image does your home carry?

If your facility hasn't developed a statement like Wesley's, you cannot turn to anything in writing to give you clarity. So where do you look? At yourself.

What do you say makes you work? A need for a paycheck? You can't get another job? Or is it a calling, a desire to care for the frail and the old and the sick?

For the answer to these questions, look into the eyes of the people you care for. Your patients will help you discover your mission.

TODAY: See what you are about.

People come to your home for different reasons. For some, their families simply can no longer provide the care they need. It is too tiring, too draining.

For others, there never were family members who cared. Once able to care for themselves, they are no longer able to pull it off. Someone discovers their situation—a small apartment or trailer, probably with no heat and/or food—and they are brought to your home.

For Mr. Hawks the circumstances were different. For almost ten years he had taken care of his wife at home. Mrs. Hawks had, to everyone's eye, Alzheimer's. Her confusion and withdrawal were complicated by dramatic changes in her physical functioning—at times she lost all control of her bowels and bladder.

Nevertheless, Mr. Hawks would take care of her, clean her and the house up, keep her safe and comfortable.

People who knew the couple's situation would say Mrs. Hawks didn't even open her eyes or talk anymore. But they never heard her husband complain.

One day Mrs. Hawks died in her bed; in less than twenty-four hours, Mr. Hawks dropped of exhaustion. He was rushed to a nursing home where relatives visiting for his wife's funeral stopped to visit. Taking one look, they knew he would not live. They said their goodbyes and left.

But, less than one year later, the wonderful staff of a southern Florida nursing home had Mr. Hawks up and running. He went back home to his avocado and lemon trees. A full five years later he was still at home.

 TODAY: Help patients go home.

The very meaning of time changes for each of us as we age, especially if we live in an institution. For staff, time passes in three blocks or shifts: days, evenings and nights.

One day the visiting chaplain was talking about the meaning of time—man's sense of time versus God's time. Florence, in her nineties, piped up, "I never know what day it is! Well, I do know that on Monday, Wednesday and Friday I get prunes!"

No longer beholden to the clock or calendar, Florence has some freedom to just relax and be. Every day can be a holiday, a birthday, a Sunday. Rather than focus on Florence's confusion, her caregivers point out that she is now living on God's or Mother Nature's time. Babies don't know if it's Monday or Tuesday either. They simply take every day as it comes, learning, loving, growing.

With this attitude Florence and the staff can concentrate on each other and the seasons, not on today's date. It's called living one day at a time, being in the present.

Loss of memory doesn't have to mean a loss of love. We can still stay close and enjoy the world around us.

TODAY: Enjoy life now.

Some people are just worriers. And some jobs cause worry.

Working in a busy long term care facility, it seems there's always something or somebody to worry or feel pressured about. Dawn, a young nurses' aide, was a worrier.

"What if I drop someone?" she would say anxiously. "What if someone accuses me of doing something I didn't do?"

Working with Dawn became a real test for some of her coworkers, especially those who got irritated with hearing Dawn's worries.

It was John, the maintenance man, who calmed Dawn down best. "Look," he said. "There's always something you could do better, faster or sooner. And there's always more to do than you have time to do. Accidents will happen. You've just got to do your best and use common sense. You're not alone. We all worry. The longer you're here, the more comfortable you'll get."

Dawn visibly relaxed after John's words. She confided that she came from a family of worriers, and that it wasn't anything she felt she could control. John laughed and told her to hang in there. "We'll help you get some control."

From that day forward, Dawn always tried to take her break so as to be around John. He made her laugh at herself. And his assurances made her feel less worried and more hopeful.

TODAY: Support your coworkers who worry.

As Shakespeare tells us, "a rose by any other word would smell as sweet." No one word can truly capture the beauty of this fragrant flower.

Nursing facilities are often given cutesy names, perhaps to make moving into one less traumatic. Golden Acres, Sunset House, Holiday House, Tranquil Haven. Sometimes, they sound like cemeteries: Everest, Golden Ridge, Happy Valley.

In fact, life inside a nursing facility is much more than the one dimensional "cute." Feelings, behaviors and actions are as varied as can be found in any small community. Only those who are uncomfortable or unfamiliar with age treat the elderly in a superficial way.

Sometimes family members will talk baby talk or talk too loud when they visit, thinking that they can't just be themselves. Something happens to people when they walk into an institution; they think they have to behave differently.

As staff members you are also good will ambassadors. Invite guests to be at ease, to act naturally. Include them in the life of the home, the daily events. The less artificial you are, the more real they will be.

You don't have to glamorize your work with old, frail people, and you don't have to put it down, either. Each day has its highs and lows, its expected and its surprises. What can be said is that inside your building there is a tiny society, teaming with life. Don't forget to remind others of this rich, full world. There's nothing simple or stereotyped about it.

TODAY: See the fullness of your world.

For those of us over thirty, it's no big deal to discover one of those stray, dark hairs sprouting out somewhere on our bodies. The same goes for moles and aches and pains: they grow with the territory.

For those of us over eighty, the discoveries and the problems are not as easy to accept, particularly when it comes to the delicate matter of going to the bathroom.

Fay, in her late eighties, was a real lady. She had been a concert pianist and had prided herself on her good grooming and impeccable appearance. However, by the time she moved into the nursing home, she had begun to lose control of her bowels and bladder.

When Linda, a nurses' aide, found Fay in her wheelchair, Fay was crying. "I couldn't get to the bathroom on time and I've messed myself," she cried quietly. Her head in her hands, she couldn't look at Linda.

"Now Fay, it's perfectly understandable," Linda said. "We're all busy around here, and I didn't check on you earlier. If you won't be angry with me for being late, I sure won't be mad at you. Taking care of you is my job. Won't you let me do my job now and get you all cleaned up?"

Linda's comforting, patient voice brought a few more tears from Fay and then a hug. "Oh dear, you are so kind. What would I do without you?" Fay said.

TODAY: Comfort your patients through the rough spots.

Why do any of us end up in this work?

I asked Alice this question one day, and she didn't miss a beat.

"That's simple," she smiled, "I took care of my grandmother and I really got into it. When she died, I came here."

Looking at the opportunities we had in our families to take care of loved ones is a pleasant exercise. We can see the gifts we received from our grandparents, our parents and sometimes even our brothers and sisters. Those gifts are of compassion, tenderness, mercy and patience. From this standpoint, the sacrifices we made in our families are no longer bitter memories of "being taken advantage of." Rather, they are sweet signposts on our journey.

Each experience with caring builds on the last. We learn from each patient and carry that new knowledge into the next room and the next day. We are made stronger and more loving with every act of caring, like a candle growing each time it is dipped into the wax.

Alice's grandmother is long gone. But the fresh chances Alice gets to show her caring nature keep her grandmother's memory alive. Alice owes part of who she is to her grandmother. And she honors her grandmother every day she comes to work.

TODAY: Honor your caring roots.

No matter how old or how rich we get, everyone likes free food. Just watch the crowds at baby showers and wedding receptions. Listen to the oohs and aahs over the snack trays and dessert table. Like kids at a fireworks display, we signal our delight over tasty treats.

This week, for no particular reason, why not bring some baked goodies to the staff lounge? Nobody has time to bake, but throwing a stick of margarine, a bag of marshmallows and four cups of crisp rice cereal on the stovetop isn't exhausting.

Cut those crispy bars up, put them in a cardboard box or coffee can (something you won't have to remember to bring home), and bring them to work.

Then have some fun watching your coworkers at break time. "How come? Why?" they will ask, munching away. Watch how this spoonful of sugar makes even the tired and grouchy perk up.

By sharing this surprise, you will tip the staff balance and change the way people talk to one another. Notice how people take their minds off of whatever is dragging them down and enjoy a bright moment. Imagine what work could be like if everyone remembered to treat each other with special treats.

TODAY: Treat the staff to treats.

Just when you think you know everything there is to know about a patient, something happens that amazes you.

That's how everyone felt about Raymond. An incredibly shy man, Raymond basically didn't speak unless spoken to. He sat most of the day wherever the staff pushed his wheelchair, gazing quietly out the window or down the hall.

Ray wasn't a difficult patient. He didn't make demands on the staff or have especially time-consuming care needs. He ate, slept, and behaved. No one seemed to visit him, and the other residents wheeled past him too. Ray didn't seem connected to anyone or anything.

One morning the activities program involved residents in reaching deep into a large plastic bag and picking out a stuffed animal.

Typically reserved, Raymond didn't even attempt to look into the sack. Instead, one of the volunteers grabbed a bright red devil, complete with horns and tail, and held it in front of him.

"Here you go, Raymond, a baby devil for you!" she said.

Raymond's face opened wide and clear, his shy expression falling away like a mask. His big smile and bright eyes stared back at the little devil as he reached out to hold it. Everyone laughed with joy, watching the animated man cradle his new creature. "Look at Raymond! He's a proud papa!" they said.

TODAY: Never give up trying to reach a quiet patient.

Tat was a Vietnamese girl who had not lived in the United States very long. She had learned enough English to get around, though few of the staff could understand her.

Starting out as a nurses' aide on nights, Tat worked silently and diligently. She moved like a graceful cat from one room to another, carefully checking on the sleeping patients, putting away their laundry, taking them to the toilet. A petite young woman, no one believed she would be able to lift and move the heavy patients. But Tat never complained and always got the job done. Working nights, there wasn't much reason to talk, so she didn't have to practice her English.

Staffing problems caused a shake up, and, after about three months on the job, Tat was transferred to the day shift. There she met up with the nursing supervisor everyone called "the bull moose."

The bull moose—given name Betty—didn't take back-talk, didn't take excuses, didn't take much of anything. And she definitely didn't take to Tat and her broken English. Whenever she could, Betty would tear into Tat, criticizing how she washed a patient, how she made the bed. "That's not how we do it in this country!" she would snarl. Tat silently took it.

One by one, the other day staff went to Tat and told her not to let Betty hurt her. They shared their own stories of abuse at Betty's hands. Everyone rallied around Tat, and built a terrific team spirit. They couldn't change Betty, but they could support one another.

TODAY: Support your shift.

Sometimes counting your blessings can be as hard as finding a four-leaf clover. Who has that kind of time?

Running around a nursing facility, always feeling you're behind, it can be particularly tough to find something good about your work.

Ann Marie, a single mother with three boys, was quick to point out what's good about being a certified nurses' aide.

"I'm not home chasing my boys!" she said. "They fight all the time and I can't take it! Working here, I put two in the day care and send one to school. Give me a patient to clean up any day!"

Some of us aren't made to take care of little children. Whatever it takes, we don't have it. Our nerves are shot by the squealing voices and high energy playtime. We choose the less active setting of a nursing facility to spend our days.

The rest of the world might not understand why we like going to work in an institution. But we know, and we're grateful for the job. We know not being at home with kids can be a blessing.

TODAY: Be grateful.

On the baseball field, the boy got into a yelling match with an umpire. The more the umpire explained his call, the fiercer the young player became. Finally, his mother called from the bleachers, "Cool it, Tommy!"

Later that night, Tommy was talking with his mom about the incident. "Mom," he said, "he sounded so much like my dad when he lectures me, and it made me madder and madder." Estranged from his father, the young man and his father had fought bitterly until Tommy left and moved to his mother's house.

"That's called 'getting plugged in,'" his mother explained. "Plugged in means the situation reminds you of another, so that you feel all the emotions you felt that other time. It can really trap you."

We all are like Tommy, with umpires who resemble our fathers. We all get plugged into people whose behaviors drive us crazy. Sometimes people just have to look like someone we had trouble with, and away we go. The trick is to recognize the pattern and learn to manage or control ourselves whenever we get triggered.

At work there are countless opportunities to get "plugged in" to people who make us upset. Other staff, residents, families and, of course, our bosses can make us steam up fast. When you get incredibly angry, more than the situation deserves, you've just been "plugged in." Stay alert for those times.

TODAY: Protect yourself from being plugged in.

May

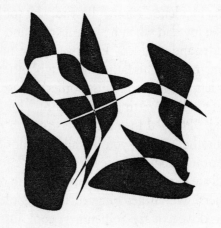

Our grandparents called it "senility." Today there are sophisticated diagnoses like Alzheimer's, Korsakoff's and related dementias. Whatever we call it, losing one's mind is never something anyone plans on in one's retirement. Still, more and more patients suffering from dementia are admitted into this country's 11,000 longterm care facilities.

Alberta was a perfect example of this population. Widowed, in her late eighties, Alberta spent most of every day telling others she needed to get to her parents' house.

"Mom is eighty-three and Dad is, well, I'm not sure," she would begin, explaining how she was responsible for preparing their evening meal. "I get up early to get to work and I bring a sandwich," she continued, enjoying the familiarity of the story. Everyone who took care of Alberta knew the tale. Once she finished the full cycle, Alberta would hastily depart, in search of a phone to call her mother.

The mind and memory are mysteries to us all. Many dementia sufferers seem to return to a time and place when they were responsible, useful, busy. Mabel was like that. She could never pause and participate in an activity.

"Didn't I tell you?" she would explain with a smile. "We're moving tomorrow! I have so much to do!"

We all know that life in an institution involves plenty of personal sacrifice and a loss of independence. It is with plenty of compassion and respect that we should care for those who have mentally escaped.

TODAY: Tend the demented with respect.

What is the message you're carrying around in the back of your mind? And how about what is in the front of your mind and even on your face?

Those messages that clutter our heads have such power over our days. Professional athletes will tell you they imagine awards ceremonies at which their skills are recognized. Dancers and musicians will concentrate on little positive expressions, sometimes called mantras, to pump up their performances.

As a career caregiver, why not consider adopting a powerful message for yourself, a personal theme song as a perpetual background sound? Carry a new tune that enlivens your day, instead of the negative thoughts that sometimes grip you, thoughts such as, "This job is too hard; the pay is too low."

King Solomon advised his people, "A happy heart is good medicine and a cheerful mind works healing." Sounds pretty good, doesn't it? Living and working from that thought will be to everyone's advantage: yours, your coworkers', and especially your patients'.

TODAY: Plant a powerful message in your mind.

So, if you ruled the world, what would it look like? Would everyone look like you, act like you, share your values and opinions? Sometimes, when we've had our fill of disagreeable people, such a fantasy seems like a good idea. At a small New England nursing home, the hiring of two male LPNs who were openly homosexual set many staff into a tail-spin.

The whispering was pretty intense, and the attacks began immediately. The most damaging act was the charge filed by a fairly new RN that both of the men had committed patient abuse. "Not once, but many times," she claimed, adding that she had proof.

Other employees listened to her angry reports and wondered why they had never witnessed either man acting abusively. Not satisfied with her informal charges, the RN went to the facility administrator.

The administrator heard the stories and then systematically called other staff in to hear their views and perceptions. At the conclusion of her investigation, she called the RN to her office.

"This is your last day of work here. We cannot handle someone with your anger and attitudes toward homosexual men on our staff. It is not anyone's job to judge someone's sexual preference. Your tactics have been nothing more than a hateful campaign to destroy two good, caring nurses. Goodbye."

The administrator then announced to the rest of the staff that, if anyone else couldn't work with individuals who were not heterosexual, they should also leave.

Life, and care, returned to normal.

TODAY: Permit others their differences.

Each shift in a nursing facility has its own character and atmosphere. Staff seem to mold to the moods, with the more high-energy, outgoing folks working days. The later the shift, the more we find more peaceful, serene employees, those who don't like big, loud group activities.

Working nights is not all quiet and harmony however. The tasks carry their share of stress and strain, and there is always something one staffer wishes another staffer would do. To comply with federal law, and often to promote good skin care, many patients must be moved or even changed at night. And, for those who have to wake a soundly sleeping patient to perform this care, it can be a real hassle.

Patients in good health and mentally alert resent being awakened in the black of night. Add the additional nuisance of having a wet diaper changed, and many patients go off the deep end. For patients who are confused or moody, this intervention is downright horrible. They will often thrash and even strike the staff, perhaps because they can't comprehend what this intruder is doing. Sometimes just placing clean laundry in the patient's drawers will lead a demented individual to believe he is being robbed.

Nurses and nurses' aides who perform awkward assignments late at night need to use the utmost tact and courtesy. Above all, they should never take negative responses personally. Continue to soothe and comfort the afflicted, seeing that it is their confusion, rather than their true feelings, which dictates their behavior.

TODAY: Deliver difficult care delicately.

For whatever reason, we all carry varying loads of insecurity around with us. Some have more self confidence than others, but just about everyone secretly worries, "Am I good enough?" More than often, we answer that question with a sad "no."

Working with, or caring for, someone with little self-esteem is a vital assignment. Above all else, we must be sensitive to the other's fragile nature. Some extra pats on the back go a long way with coworkers who have spent much of their life being put down or wondering if they are of any value. As an outsider, you are in a perfect position to observe their work and praise it.

Individuals who don't feel good about themselves don't always act as though they are no good. Sometimes people with little confidence will present themselves as super certain and even bossy. Don't be fooled. The more they "know it all," the more likely they are full of self-doubt.

Patients can be equally uncertain and depressed by a sense of little personal worth. Again, as the outsider, you can assume the delicious task of turning these folks on to their own greatness. Not only do they have a lifetime to be proud of, but they are permitting you the opportunity to take care of them. Without patients, caregivers don't exist.

TODAY: Help someone feel good about herself.

Dotty lived in the nursing home with two other room-mates. One was always complaining. Nothing ever satisfied Rita.

One day, while Dotty was talking with a visitor, Rita began her tirade against a staff person. When she didn't let up, Dotty and her visitor moved out to the sunroom at the end of the hall.

"Doesn't that drive you crazy? What do you think of all of those complaints?" the visitor asked.

"None of my business," Dotty replied matter-of-factly. This healthy attitude kept Dotty from being pulled down into Rita's badlands.

Dotty's motto "none of my business" can keep all of us out of nasty situations that do nothing but trouble us. It's a second cousin to another bit of folk wisdom, this one shared by Doris, a nurses' aide.

"One of the best ways I've found to deal with an angry person is to simply bite my tongue," said Doris one day, after describing her encounter with Rita.

"Sometimes people just need to complain. They don't want any suggestions or even a response. They just need to talk. So, even though I have plenty I could say, I just bite my tongue."

TODAY: Mind your business and bite your tongue.

In her novel *As We Are Now,* May Sarton portrays a woman's final days in a small country home for the infirm. The one bright spot at the otherwise dreary place is an aide named Anna.

Have I ever before really understood the power and healing grace of sensitive hands like Anna's? Have I ever experienced loving as I do in one glance from her amazing clear eyes that take in at once what my needs are, whether it be food or a gentle caress, a pillowcase changed, a glass of warm milk? No wonder so many old men fall in love with their nurses! I used to think of them with contempt—old babies, old self-indulgent babies. And now here I am in much the same plight!

This book was recommended to me by a nurses' aide at Vernon Green. She suggested I read it, stating that *As We Are Now* was the very reason she was doing this work.

"I don't wonder if I am important, or if I am making a difference," she explained.

Each day, little books lie unread by us. Sweet little books lying in the beds of our facilities, with old wrinkled faces waiting for us to stop and read. Their stories are like May Sarton's—about the power and grace of your healing hands.

TODAY: Read the faces around you.

Just when you think you can take no more, along comes more.

This was precisely the case in a rural facility that had been operating short-staffed for more than a year. No one stayed with the Director of Nursing job. At last count, four people had tried the job in the last eighteen months. The administrator was now doubling as the director of nursing, and the wear and tear was visible.

This was not the best setting for the news that one of the charge nurses had been diagnosed with extensive, inoperable breast and bone cancer. Who had any more compassion to give? Where would they find the energy to care about yet one more hurting person?

Still, as befit the stunning beauty of human beings, the staff reached deep into their souls and found yet more love to give. Carol, the sick staffer, became the rallying point for staff and residents. The activities staff organized card- and bread-making parties, making sure something was delivered to Carol from the home at least weekly. Social Services even arranged for staff and resident visits to Carol's house. Flowering plants grown at the nursing home were brought in.

Each day, it seemed, someone thought of Carol in a new way. In a short period of time, the focus was no longer on the staffing problems of the institution, but on their loved one, Carol. Having a sick person on staff had brought renewed vigor and the spirit of kindness. Carol proved to be a precious reminder to all of their reason for being.

TODAY: Let weakness make you strong.

T-shirts and bumper stickers are not the only way we can shout our one-liners at the world.

Just visit any Chinese restaurant and check out the fortune cookies. No matter how many cookies we've had, or how old we are, we always hope for the ideal message. A recent cookie held this pearl: "Your heart will always make itself known through your words."

How honest and healthy is your heart? Your words will give you a big clue. When you see a coworker having an especially bad day, what do you usually do? Ignore her? Tell someone else? Criticize or report her?

A loving heart directs us to go to the staffer who is not her regular self. "You're not yourself today, Margaret. Do you need a break? Are you sick or tired? Can I help you?"

Margaret may not have even noticed she was being abrupt and mean with the residents. She might not have realized her problems at home had spilled into the workplace. Your tender concern can help her get a grip.

Sure it's easier, and juicier, to gossip with others about how nasty Margaret is being, but does that make things better? Deep down, your heart is full of love and mercy for others. Make sure you speak those words when someone is having a bad day. Ask your coworkers to promise to let you know when they're having a bad day. You're all in this together.

TODAY: Make your heart known through your words.

Nobody plans on getting so old and sick that they spend all their money and must go on welfare. Yet more than half the patients in nursing homes across the United States are in precisely this situation.

Those who have relied upon the welfare system during difficult times know the monthly payments are small. Imagine how thinly these dollars are spread for nursing home care.

Your patients are proud people who undoubtedly worked hard all their lives. Many refused welfare or government support their whole working lives, even when widowed with children. Today they cannot pay their bill for nursing care. Some may not even realize their way is being paid for by the welfare program.

As a caregiver, what is important to you is not how people pay for their care, or even how much. Whether they are independently wealthy and able to pay the bill, or rely upon tax dollars, it makes no difference. In fact the less you know about who pays what, the freer you are to simply care without distinctions.

Human nature often makes us more respectful of those with money. Age and disability are the great levelers. Wealth buys the same bed as welfare. And now is the time for you to serve all of your patients equally and tenderly.

TODAY: Care for all equally.

Mother's Day falls this time of year. And so does National Nursing Home Week.

It's no accident that the week of celebration kicks off on the big day we recognize moms. After all, moms are the ultimate caregivers. There's no tougher job than being a mom, except perhaps being a nurses' aide.

How many of your patients will be remembered by someone on Mother's Day? How many will get a card, a call, a visit? How many never had children?

This can be such a tough day for women. Patients who have outlived some or all of their children can get very blue and even withdrawn, looking back on the death of a child. Women who gave up children for adoption or ended a pregnancy can also be haunted by decisions made long ago. Still others can feel guilty about being too strict, or not strict enough.

Help your patients handle whatever reaction or feelings they have about this day. Listen to them and, if it feels right, share with them your experience of the day.

TODAY: Be sensitive to mothers.

Like schools, nursing facilities have set routines. At 7 a.m. people are getting out of bed. At 7 p.m. people are getting back into bed. So goes the day, full of predictable rituals and tasks.

Perhaps that's one of the reasons a performance by live musicians is so welcome in such settings. Just when everyone is at the point of screaming at the same old monotonous music filling the building, faces get soft, curious, content.

Such was the case one hot Sunday afternoon in June when four student cellists, aged ten to twelve, held a recital in the activities room. Accompanied by their teacher on the piano, the young musicians drew an ever-growing crowd. At the top of the program, around 2 p.m., there were about fifteen people in the room. By the end, almost double that number had peeked or wandered in.

The lemonade and cookies that followed were the perfect touch, increasing this feeling of a pleasant treat. Even more folks peeked or wandered in for the refreshments.

But the biggest treat was yet to come. The cello teacher's mother-in-law, who had recently moved into the facility, was urged to play the piano for the audience. A gracious woman in her late eighties, the pianist at first demurred. "Why, I haven't practiced!" she said, adding in a whisper, "That's always been a good excuse!"

At last she sat at the grand piano and played a Chopin etude flawlessly from memory. The listeners were captivated; several were crying. Upon further prompting, this lovely lady serenaded the room with Debussy's "Reverie," again from memory.

Following the applause, and more prompting, the pianist said she thought she had a Chopin etude she could play. And she did, the same one she had played a few minutes earlier. Upon finishing, her daughter-in-law suggested another piece, and again she performed Debussy's "Reverie." Totally unaware she had performed either piece twice, she delivered precious, perfect renditions each time. And each time there were even fewer dry eyes in the room. The applause was mighty.

TODAY: Treasure inner beauty.

As most mothers know, it's hard to be too careful when trying to guard against accidents. And, as most staff in a healthcare facility know, accidents happen.

What happened that morning right across from the nurses' station was not an accident anyone had even considered. After all, the patients were sick, old and frail. Staff had been instructed to guard against many kinds of incidents, but who would have imagined attempted rape? After the horrifying event was over, the staff sat around a table with the administrator trying to reconstruct how it had happened.

It seems Alice was in the middle stages of Alzheimer's disease. She no longer knew what was socially unacceptable behavior. She frequently walked around the nursing home holding her skirt up, sometimes pulling it above her head. As is the case in most facilities, after the first few displays the staff mentally filed Alice's behavior into their daily experience. Very matter of factly, they would pull Alice's skirt back down, reminding her that she should not pull it up. Everyone knew Alice couldn't remember, so they just added "pull Alice's skirt down" to their list of things to do.

Bernard was a mysterious patient. His diagnosis was less clear. Everyone did know that he was grumpy, withdrawn and unpleasant—the kind of guy staff didn't get close to easily.

And while the staff had long ago stopped noting Alice's daily panty flashes as important, Bernard had obviously taken her gesture as a come-on, a tease. When he forced himself on bewildered Alice, whose room was right across from the nurses' station, Bernard basically felt he had been invited. "She was flaunting it!" he yelled, as frantic staff pulled him out of the room.

Clearly there weren't enough staff to have someone stay with Alice or Bernard twenty-four hours a day. What could be done?

Further discussion led the staff to realize that, if Alice could no longer wear a skirt appropriately, she shouldn't be dressed in one. From that day forward, Alice wore pants, a simple change which provided much greater protection. In-services were planned on preventive measures as well as patient sexuality.

TODAY: Remember your patients are still men and women.

Looking back on our behavior or job performance, we can sometimes beat ourselves up for an inferior effort. Sometimes we can make ourselves feel pretty guilty for not doing enough or doing it poorly. Other times our tempers or anger might even make us abusive.

When the wave of self-recognition and self-loathing takes over, it is not the time to beat yourself up. Honestly reflecting on your work is healthy. Seeing how far you've come and grown is healthy. You can even rejoice that actions you once took without thinking are no longer acceptable to you.

Abraham Lincoln, an American hero, a man whom many consider close to perfect, did not indulge in second guessing. He had to make tough decisions, historic decisions which so divided this nation that young men took sides, fought and died by the tens of thousands. Speaking of his approach to life, Lincoln wrote some wise words that can guide us all today: "I have simply tried to do what seemed best each day, as each day came."

Sounds so basic, doesn't it? And yet we all know that much of our thinking can easily focus on regrets about the past or worries about the future. Being in the present is not an easy assignment. Yet if President Lincoln could do it, we can work toward living by this guiding philosophy too.

TODAY: Do your best.

The hospice movement is an old European approach to care for the dying. In the United States, hospice programs have been primarily the domain of home health agencies. Recently nursing homes too have begun to develop hospice programs. Staff and/or volunteers are trained in this tender way of being with terminally ill patients and their families. The object is to provide the patient with a pain free, comfortable situation, and the family—if they wish—with plenty of attention and opportunities for involvement.

The root of the word "hospice" is Greek, and its literal translation speaks volumes. Hospice means both "guest" and "host."

There is no one English word that conveys the concept of being both the served and the server. The beauty of hospice, then, is that, in providing merciful attention to the dying patient, the caregiver reaps many benefits as well. This sense of giving and receiving can apply to the broad category of caregiving too.

Caregivers often refer to rewards of the heart. When people question how anyone could work daily around the sick and the dying ("Isn't it depressing?" they ask), caregivers shake their heads "no."

No-strings-attached caring means no one is sure where the host ends and the guest begins. Both parties feel they are receiving more than they are giving. Such is the beauty of caring.

TODAY: Be guest and host.

Who knows what the insurance adjuster first said when he read the claim? Reported by a harried nursing home administrator, the insurance form went something like this:

Our brand new $12,000 photocopier was too big to get through the doorway of the business office, so it was temporarily set up in the hall. The maintenance man was going to remove the door and trim to move it in to the office tomorrow. Sometime during the night, a confused male resident saw the large white object with a bin on the side and mistook it for a urinal. Our machine is no longer working. We believe the electrical panel was ruined.

If you don't laugh, you'll cry, right? The line between the comedy and the tragedy of the event is so faint, who's to say what is the proper reaction?

Working with confused, often seriously mentally ill patients, one never knows precisely what to expect. Like the facility that had a former professional pickpocket move in. Every night at bedtime, sensitive staff had to respectfully help the confused gentleman undress, collecting all the cigarette lighters, combs, pens and the like from his pockets and returning them to their rightful owners. Laugh or cry?

Staff who celebrate their tenth and even twentieth anniversaries as caregivers have learned to survive and even enjoy the unexpected. Laughing is part of their secret.

TODAY: Laugh with love.

Watching the administrator of a nursing facility sit in his beautifully decorated office, writing memos and making decisions, direct care providers can feel pretty put out.

"What does he know about taking care of these patients? He's got it easy! Let him come and try to get ten patients up and dressed this morning!"

Judging someone else's job is not only foolhardy, it's plain dangerous. First of all, unless you've done the job there's no way you can fully understand the pressures.

For instance, if the administrator isn't the owner, he or she must answer to an owner who is very interested in the bottom line. And if he or she is the owner, there are concerns about family investment and stability, particularly if the business was started by his or her parents.

Indulging in this tempting habit of putting down management, workers start to wear away that critical feeling of team. If a mother tears down her husband to the kids, how does that help the family? Once respect is lost, the bottom falls out on any team or relationship.

Participating in this destructive habit, caregivers also open up the possibility of turnabout—administrators unfairly minimizing the role of direct care staff. Once the route is opened up for such travel, it easily becomes a two way street.

Why not learn more about all the administration does to keep the facility open and running smoothly? Why not devote a little energy to talking to management, instead of about it? You're all part of the big body called nursing home, whether you're the hands, feet, voice or mind.

 TODAY: Appreciate the administration.

On Thursdays or Fridays, or whatever day is payday, that dollar figure on your check can be pretty discouraging, especially living in this culture in which we want to measure people based on what they wear, drive and live in.

Having our hourly wage dictate our worth is a crazy way to live. Just look at the patients in your facility. Does their personal wealth mean much to you? You get to know them purely on their personalities, not their purses.

Helen Keller, the famous blind, deaf and mute author, could not see what people wore, drove or lived in. She wrote: "The best and most beautiful things in the world cannot be seen or touched, but are felt in the heart."

Robbed of her senses of sight and sound, as well as speech, Helen Keller couldn't be distracted by glitz. Money probably didn't mean much to her or have much power over her.

For Ruby, a nurses' aide for thirty-nine years, her wages went beyond the form of weekly paychecks. "I like the unexpected thank you's," Ruby explained, recalling the appreciation expressed by a patient she didn't even know could talk.

Patty, a younger aide, put it this way: "I like giving happiness." Clearly, no paycheck can equal her satisfaction.

TODAY: Write your own paycheck.

Everything on earth has its cycles, its seasons. Snakes shed their skins, tadpoles their tails, babies leave their bottles behind.

For women, many of us experience the less welcome cycle of PMS (premenstrual syndrome) or PMT (premenstrual tension).

Stephanie DeGraff Bender, a noted author and health educator, has stated that PMS is not in your head: it's definitely a physical problem. It can damage your self-esteem, relationships and career. The good news is that it can be treated.

Like any problem that clouds our thinking or acting, PMS treatment isn't one magic pill and pouf! it's gone. Mrs. Bender points out in her books *PMS: A Positive Program to Gain Control* and *PMS: Questions and Answers* (published by Price Stern Sloan) that the depression, anger and anxiety associated with PMS require several different approaches.

Diet, exercise and hormones all greatly affect the guilt, embarrassment and other bad feelings that arise with PMS. And perhaps more than any other remedy, becoming aware of this cycle in your life can give you some immediate relief. Talk to other women, especially those in your own family. Ask them if they have experienced what you're going through.

If certain behaviors and statements only trigger you at certain times of the month, you may have PMS. Why is it that a forgetful husband is easily forgiven during days one through twenty-one, but is cut no slack in days twenty-one to twenty-eight? Why can a repetitive patient be cute, and even funny, early in your cycle, but make you a crazy woman later on?

Make a pact with some coworkers. Learn more about PMS, its causes and treatment.

P.S. Male staff—don't think this knowledge isn't for you! Not knowing may be hazardous to your health!

TODAY: Learn about PMS.

Every so often the news will carry the grisly story of a young mother who has suffocated, abandoned or otherwise killed her baby.

We all cringe at such reports, imagining the totally vulnerable infant at the mercy of a troubled parent. Confronted with the responsibility of a 100 percent helpless child, the mother snaps. As bystanders, we wonder how could anyone, especially a blood relation, so abuse trust.

Trust is an essential ingredient in the makeup of any decent caregiver. Brett, a young nurses' aide, summed up his sense of the job this way: "They trust me." He saw the weight of that trust as mighty, a heavy responsibility for him to uphold.

Often, like helpless babies, the frail, bedridden elderly are at the will of their "keepers." Frequently alone in a room with an employee, who sees the cruel pinches or hears the cutting remarks?

Deep within each human being there is an ethical rudder that keeps the individual upright and right on. Brett was in touch with his, seeing just how incredibly powerful he was in the lives of his patients. Paying attention to that rudder, Brett is far less likely to hurt those placed in his care. He does, in effect, earn the patients' trust on an ongoing basis.

TODAY: Earn your patients' trust.

Roy is a wise man. He has lived a long, active life, raised two children, outlived two wives, and left a mark in his chosen profession of wildlife management.

I asked Roy, in his ninth decade, about his philosophy of life. This is in part what he wrote me:

> A wise person stated that the human body was a fit engine for the human soul. We must give it good care in order to exist. I am going to try to streamline and get rid of handicaps. It is good to know that if we do our very best, letting our past guide us and our wisdom and faith show us how, that is where our responsibilities end and the higher powers take it from there.

How many of us can truly call our bodies fit engines? I remember Toni, a restaurant manger, who was hosting a meeting of nurses. "Are these women really all nurses?" she asked incredulously. "I've never had so many smokers in one room!"

For the tense, overworked healthcare worker, a cigarette break is a welcome moment. But breaks don't have to be tied to a cigarette. And as more and more research is generated about the deadly power of cigarettes and their smoke, the smoke-free break seems smarter and smarter.

In Vermont, smoking is now prohibited in all public places, including the common areas of nursing homes. For some caregivers, this law meant a major lifestyle change. It has become an opportunity to do what they've been talking about for a long time: quit. Or, as Roy suggests about our health, "We must give it good care in order to exist."

TODAY: Keep your engine fit.

Division of labor makes a lot of sense. Henry Ford perfected this practice with his assembly line for the manufacturing of automobiles. Every worker had a job and a station, with none duplicating the other. Working with machines, such rigid job descriptions make plenty of sense.

When your product is not cars or widgets but health care, strict enforcement of who does what isn't as cut and dried. Especially when the patients are confused and can't tell a laundry worker from a nurses' aide from a housekeeper.

Some people might think that having looser job-descriptions would cause chaos. In reality, flexibility can be the positive net-result. But for the looser team approach to work, all employees must see the need for, and value of, pitching in when needed.

Martha was a registered nurse. Once an aide, she had returned to school and worked for many years to earn her nursing license. Given this arduous struggle, Martha was not about to do any work that others would label "aide's duties."

When a resident urinated on the lobby linoleum, Martha excused herself and went off to find an aide. Fifteen minutes later she returned with a harried aide who took a paper towel and cleaned up the mess in five seconds. It was at that moment that a naive visitor asked, "Martha, don't you know how to clean up a spill?" At that moment Martha got it. She saw the silly situation her rigid thinking had caused.

"No, I was thinking that cleaning wasn't an RN's job. But I could have handled it fifteen minutes ago and let the aide finish her work!"

TODAY: Pitch in when you're needed.

∽

The weather can be such a bummer. No matter how well you've planned your picnic, nobody can control the rain. Some of us find such powerful forces in our lives totally unfair, and we expend lots of energy whining about the raw deal we got.

Ingrid was the grand dame of this brand of power whining. The less control she had, the more she whined about the unfairness of it all. If she had to work overtime, she complained she was being taken advantage of. If she didn't work overtime, she complained others were making extra money when she wasn't. Ingrid couldn't be pleased. She sure could be ticked off.

Listening to Ingrid's constant whining about circumstances beyond her control, Carol finally couldn't take it anymore. She remembered something a high school teacher had written on the blackboard when his pupils were protesting the grading curve.

In the break room, Ingrid was carrying on about how unfair it was that her sister got her mail at 10:30 every morning, but it didn't get delivered to Ingrid's house till after 3. Carol jumped up and ran to the blackboard. She wrote "So what?"

"Ingrid," Carol said, "That's what I have to say about your complaints that are against forces out of your control. So what, I don't wish to be mean, but my point is… (here Carol stopped talking and wrote on the black board) What's so."

"That's just 'what's so,' Ingrid. So let it go, and talk about things you have some influence over."

TODAY: Look for "so what's" in your day.

When the patients who now live in nursing homes were born eighty-five or ninety years ago, they were born at home. By the time they had children, hospital births were becoming common. Now almost everyone reading this book was born in a hospital.

Health care is constantly evolving, changing, growing to better meet the ever-changing needs of its customers. Nursing homes, once the homes of many kinds of elderly people with a variety of diagnoses, are fast becoming mental-health facilities where confused and demented men and women finish out their days.

For the family members who visit these senile loved ones, the time together can be bittersweet. Rarely able to make an emotional connection with their mother or father, the visiting relative must be satisfied with feeding or walking this "stranger." The feelings of isolation and abandonment can be significant.

Sensing this loss of companionship and increase in frustration, one nursing home staff brainstormed about how to make the visit to their facility more meaningful. It was the cook who had the idea. "Why don't we ask our visitors to deliver the dinner meals we prepare for shut-ins in the area? We have not been able to find a regular volunteer driver."

Now, visitors to this facility routinely stop by the kitchen and ask "Anything I can drop off on my way home?" Quite often a meal or snack is waiting for a homebound elder in the community.

TODAY: Promote connections between people.

In our culture, when you aren't earning a living, working a job or even able to take care of yourself, it is pretty easy to decide you're not worth much. A young hospice patient once told a volunteer, "When the nurses come to see me, I think they're just waiting for me to die."

Feeling useful is vital to our sense of well-being. And we can't just pretend we are useful; it must be real.

That's what was so beautiful about the simple project the chaplain organized one Friday morning during the facility's weekly nondenominational worship service.

The chaplain's teenage son had finally cleaned his room, and among the discards was a bushel basket of stuffed animals. Many won at the fair, the little creatures were still in good shape. That Friday, the nursing facility worshipers were asked to pick an animal from the basket.

"This is your animal," the chaplain explained, "to love and hold as long as you want. If at some time you feel you have given it enough love and would like to give it away, let me know."

A mission project had been set up to send toy animals to children in the former Soviet Union, and the chaplain said she would make sure their donations got shipped.

At the end of the service, about ten of the twenty-five residents signed little cards and placed them with their critter in a box bound for Russia.

The remaining fifteen residents wheeled contentedly back to their rooms with a new object to love perched in their laps.

TODAY: Remind patients they can give.

Ask anyone who hires people—what is one of the most important qualities in a good employee? Reliability.

Being reliable means you get to work on time, that people can count on you. It means you don't make a lot of call-ins or excuses, but that you are job-ready. When so many patients depend on so few staff, being on time is even more critical. After all, your tardiness probably means someone doesn't have his or her basic needs met—like getting to the bathroom on time.

Marie had been late all her life. Other than her birth at 3 a.m., Marie joked she had never gotten out of bed early. But all joking aside, her chronic tardiness was way beyond amusing. It was downright disgusting. Marie no longer kept track of how many jobs she had lost because of this problem. Why would she want to recall these statistics anyway?

Like an alcoholic who always has a reason for a drink, Marie had a limitless set of stories to cover her lateness. Traffic, children, engines, sickness—the list was endless. No longer able to hold a job, Marie was working for a nursing agency that sent her out as a temporary floor-nurse when employers called. She still came late, but the short-staffed facility was so happy to see her that her tardiness was rarely mentioned!

A perfect scam to keep her racket going? Not so. Marie longed for stability in her life, for a good benefits package, for a retirement plan, and most of all, for a feeling of belonging. But without facing her bad habits, she would continue to drift.

TODAY: Face your bad habits.

In college they're called night owls—those kids who seem to come alive with the theme song of the Tonight Show. They stay up all night and even organize their class schedules so they can sleep until 2 p.m.

In the nursing facility, residents who like the night-life are clearly the exception, not the rule. Most folks are content to get their pajamas on soon after they finish eating. By 7 p.m. the halls are usually pretty empty.

But what about our old night owls? Those folks who always watched the late movie, stayed up and did jigsaw puzzles, or finished a good mystery novel? What happens to them in the regimented lifestyle of an institution?

If caregivers are creative, plenty! One Connecticut facility has devoted an entire wing to the "Leno-Letterman" crowd. An activities assistant works the late shift, makes popcorn and stages marvelous film festivals. Cooking and art projects go on into the wee hours, until the residents decide the day is finally over.

When bedtime comes, because they are segregated in a separate wing, nobody makes noise and disturbs the sleeping. Formally diagnosed with a disorder known as "sun-downers," these residents are comfortable and well cared for. The wise staff of the facility built a program to serve the people, rather than force the people to fit the program.

TODAY: Create options for special residents.

The story goes that a building contractor wanted to take his very patient wife on a three-month tour of Europe. Having foregone vacations for years when he was just too busy to leave, the contractor was nearing retirement.

"I am taking my wife on a long overdue trip," he told his head foreman, Jim. "While I am gone, I would like you to build me her dream house. Here are the plans, and here is my bank book. Spend whatever you need to make the house a show-piece. I've worked with you a long time, Jim, and I trust you."

So the stunned foreman began the project. Not three days went by before Jim was placing his first supply order. "What grade of lumber do you want?" the clerk asked. "Oh, an unfinished grade will do," Jim said. And so Jim began his practice of withdrawing top dollar from the bank account, buying seconds, and pocketing the difference. When his boss returned, Jim toured him through the gorgeous home. And while he had cut many corners, using the cheapest supplies whenever possible, no such shortcomings were visible. Jim had planned carefully.

"Jim," his grateful boss said, "I didn't tell you when I left, because I wanted to make this a surprise." Handing Jim the front door key he said, "This is your house. My 'thank you' for being such a loyal, trustworthy employee."

The moral of the story is an obvious one. As the Chinese say, "What goes out the door comes back through the window." You get what you give.

Make sure you deal with everyone, from residents to coworkers, to visitors, to survey nurses, in the same even, and considerate way. No one deserves anything less. And who knows? That frog could just be a prince.

TODAY: Live the Golden Rule.

Those of us who argue with our children about what movies they are permitted to watch or rent know that defining quality and pornography is a tough assignment.

In the workplace, trying to figure out what is a great joke and what is sexual harassment can be equally confounding. After all, isn't the eye and ear of the beholder what really counts?

Working in a primarily female profession (with most of the patients women as well) nursing facility staff may experience an uncommon kind of sexual harassment. Instead of the typical problem where men bother women, the nursing facility can become the site of women harassing men. Unknowingly, groups of female employees can tease new or young male employees beyond the point of humor. Telling a man he has "nice buns" or asking if he has a hairy chest can seem harmless to the questioner but humiliating to the questioned.

The fellowship of females can often create a false atmosphere in which basic courtesies toward men can be forgotten or neglected. Make sure this gang mentality doesn't contaminate your home. Sexual harassment goes both ways.

TODAY: Be aware of sexual harassment.

So what will your obituary say? Will it describe your family? Hobbies? Education? The older we get, the more this question pops up. Just what will your life have meant?

Determined to recognize the incredible achievement of living a hundred years, we started Centenarians of Vermont, an honorary society for citizens one hundred years of age and older. To our amazement, no one else was honoring them.

By informing doctors, home health agencies, senior centers and, of course, nursing homes, we put the word out: calling all hundred-year-olds and older!

The response has been glorious. More than sixty-five Vermonters have been identified as eligible for initiation into the society. An engraved pin and welcoming letter is sent to each new member. Vermont's Governor and the president of the United States are informed of the inductee and they send letters of congratulations.

The daughter of one new member wrote the Society following her mother's initiation. "You can't imagine how much this has meant to mother. She hasn't gotten any mail addressed to her personally in close to 10 years. We've hung your letter in a frame above her chair. She asks everyone to read it when they drop over. Thank you for honoring her."

To think a letter from a stranger could mean so much! Why not start a Centenarian chapter in your state?

TODAY: Honor the old among you.

Memorial Day falls at the end of this month. For some Americans, it simply means that the banks are closed, that mail isn't delivered, and they may have the day off. For healthcare workers, especially those working in old soldiers' homes, the Memorial Day holiday can be a high-energy event. Some of your patients may even be in your care because of injuries or problems related to military life. Others may have their care paid for by the US Government.

Veterans' healthcare facilities are unique in that they generally have a much higher percentage of male employees and male residents. The prevalence of substance abuse histories is also higher. Unions are more likely to represent employees, as the facility is usually government owned. And at least one report indicates that another unique aspect of veterans' homes is that patient-abuse reports are greater than the average.

We can understand most of these variables, but why the abuse statistic? Common sense would suggest that "old soldiers never die," that they continue to be aggressive to the end. Traditionally, males of the species have been the fighters, the ones who settle conflict physically. After all, the American family stereotype has been "wait till your father gets home."

Knowing all these distinctions, caregivers need to be sensitive to the sometimes special needs of male patients. We cannot generalize concerning an entire sex, but collecting information about common traits and qualities is just plain smart when our business is people. While our patients might not even be aware of these dynamics, good direct-care providers can adjust accordingly and actually prevent confrontations.

TODAY: Resolve conflict peacefully.

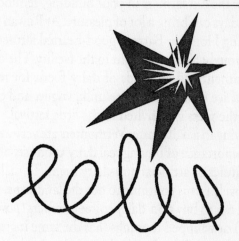

June

June 1

All across this country June is dairy month and has been for decades. On farms there is plenty to cheer about come June. Cows are back in the pastures grazing on new grass, milk production jumps up from the winter output, and calves are being born.

For the old farmers in your building, reminders of dairy days can bring a lot of pleasure. At Rowan Court Nursing Home in Barre, a good-hearted farmer actually brought a real cow right to the facility. The dietary department had all kinds of dairy foods for refreshments: ice cream, chocolate milk, yogurt and cheese. Even the press was invited to the little festival.

Living in a dairy state, Vermonters are very aware of the importance of buying real dairy products only, no substitutes or artificial non-dairy items. To make sure our lovely farms continue to dot the landscape, we are asked not to buy non-dairy coffee creamers (powdered paint) or whipped toppings (has the same ingredients as antifreeze). Buy the real thing; help your health and the economy's health.

TODAY: Observe June as Dairy Month.

One of the hazards of large group living is that, too often, one size must fit all. Patients aren't generally encouraged or even permitted to choose their bed times or what and when they want to eat. For the sake of order and convenience, many decisions are made by others.

Students in college dorms often complain of similar constraints. "No nails in the walls," the rule states. "No stereos after midnight." Eventually, such rules provoke most young people into finding their own apartments before graduation.

For the residents of nursing facilities, the chances are pretty remote that they will seek and find their freedom living "off campus." Life is to be lived and completed in the institution.

Greek legend tells the story of Procrustes, a highway bandit who invited his victims to a fatal sleep. Procrustes may have promoted himself and his bed as user-friendly; unlike the standardized beds of other hostelries, his bed would fit each of his "guests" perfectly!

But what guests didn't learn until they arrived at Procrustes' establishment was that it took some sadistic action to make the accommodations fit. The short vicims had their legs stretched on the rack until they fit the bed perfectly. As for the tall victims, Procrustes simply chopped off a part of each leg. A perfect fit!

The analogy to institutional life is obvious. We can do some pretty damaging things to our residents to make them fit our programs and buildings and rules. The more timid, tired, polite or depressed a resident is, the more staff can be manipulative and force them to "go along to get along." But is that what being a guest in your facility is really about?

TODAY: Adjust programs, not people.

Our children are teaching us a lot about caring for the environment. In my home our son pushed recycling until finally we made a commitment to sort and return all of our glass, cans, plastic, paper and cardboard. To be honest, we had gotten sloppy and blind to our bad habits. We said we didn't pollute, but by dumping everything at the landfill we were actually polluters.

Hidden pollution is common in most nursing facilities, and for the same reason. We become used to our jobs and habits and no longer question or think about what we could do to improve and protect the environment. It often takes someone with a new outlook, such as our children or a visitor, to wake us up.

In one old three story facility, a workshop leader was scheduled to train staff for three hours in a small meeting room. Unfamiliar with the building, the instructor set up her portable flip chart, arranged her handouts at the table and began her presentation.

Not ten minutes into her program, the wall intercom amplified this announcement: "Susan Peabody, you have a call on line one. Susan Peabody, pick up line one." While the workshop participants seemed undisturbed by the announcement, the visiting leader was clearly rattled. She collected her thoughts and continued. Less than two minutes later another broadcast was made: "Attention residents! There will be a sing-along on A Wing in ten minutes. Please come to the sing-along on A wing."

This time, while her students continued to be undisturbed by the interruption, the leader was fuming.

"This place is like O'Hare Airport! Do you have those kinds of announcements all day long?"

The class said yes, many looking at one another as if to say, "What's her problem?"

The leader then put aside her prepared workshop and began to educate the staff on the subject of Noise Pollution. Reminding them that this was a home, not just a place of work, she began to sensitize the employees about the disorientation such constant booming voices cause. She recalled the story of the resident sitting alone near a nursing station when a male voice floated through the air, "Is anyone at the nurses' station?" The frightened resident answered, "Is that you, God?"

Studies have shown the majority of paging done in nursing facilities is for personal calls. Whose comfort and well-being are such policies designed to serve? Staff or residents?

TODAY: Reduce noise pollution.

In 1917 the United States was full of orphanages. More common than homes for the aging, orphanages took care of children whose parents died from the great flu epidemic and other untreatable diseases. The children of unwed mothers were also keeping such institutions full.

In reviewing the deaths in the country's orphanages, a team of doctors and nurses discovered that babies admitted before they had reached the age of one usually died. In fact, as incredible as it seems, the death rate for infants under the age of one in the nation's orphanages was 100 percent! Faced with this horrifying reality, the medical team began to research what other countries did to care for infant orphans.

Their investigation produced this fact: in Dusseldorf, Germany, at an orphanage attached to the city hospital, babies did not die. After much deliberation the team decided to travel (by steamship) to Germany to learn why the Dusseldorf care was superior.

Once at the orphanage the Americans carefully observed the care, studying every variable they could identify. What was the temperature of the rooms? How often were children taken outside? How many babies to a room? The diet? Medicine?

After nearly two weeks the American visitors and their German counterparts met for one last session. The Americans were clearly disappointed. "We've learned nothing," they said. "Maybe the German diet is a little different, but basically we do what you do."

At that moment, across the back of the room, a small, old woman walked by quietly holding a baby.

"Who's that?" an American doctor asked.

Looking over, an orphanage staff member said, "Oh, that's old Anna."

"Does she work here?"

"Yes."

The American doctor became impatient. "Well, we asked to meet with all your staff. Why didn't we talk with her?"

"She's just a housekeeper," the German official explained.

"Then why is she holding a baby?" the American persisted.

"Well, when we have a baby who is failing to thrive, who is not responding to anything we have tried, we give it to old Anna. And she holds it. And somehow it lives," the German said.

Old Anna and her love was the secret to life itself in the Dusseldorf orphanage. Your tender loving touch is equally powerful.

TODAY: Touch your patients lovingly.

Are you a Lone Ranger? "I can do it myself." "I don't need your help." "It's just easier to do it alone."

A noted New England therapist, working with nurses' aides returning to work after being seriously injured on the job, spoke of their great devotion to their work:

> Some of them get hurt because, when a very big patient starts to fall, they try to stop her or hold her all alone. They are so devoted to the patient, they don't think of their own well-being.

While nursing facilities are certainly not known for an overabundance of staff, trying to do tough lifting or transferring patients alone can be downright hazardous. Working as a team, two or more staff can minimize the potential for injury and accidents.

Being in partnership with others is an art. Sometimes it takes more time not to work alone and, instead, to develop a working relationship with others, but this approach has value beyond just physical safety.

Family members who regularly visit facilities can become "partners in care" working with the staff on the care plan for their loved one. Rather than seeing the meddling mother of a severely brain-injured teenager as a nuisance, the smart staff builds her into their plan. With a little instruction, the mom can wash her son, feed him, even get him ready for bed. She so desperately wants to connect with her son, and staff sure can use some help.

Alert residents at Pleasant Manor Nursing Center took it upon themselves to help orient and direct their confused roommates and other demented residents of the facility. While functioning as guides, not as guards, the helping residents worked hard to prevent others from taking things that weren't theirs, wandering into dangerous situations or leaving the buildings. Closely coordinated with the staff, these caring residents made everyone's life at the Manor truly more Pleasant.

TODAY: Make some partnerships.

Memorial services are grand programs. Often the activities department organizes them, but anyone on staff can take the lead position.

At Berlin Health and Rehabilitation Center, the activities staff realized that in the first six months of the year more than twenty residents had died. It was decided to have some kind of service to remember them.

A list of the dead residents was circulated among the staff and everyone was asked to jot down their memories. Families and other residents were also invited to share memories and attend the service. Blue and white ribbons were made to pin on all those who attended, and candles were put on the altar table.

At the ceremony, as each deceased resident's name was read, the activities director read the memories she had collected. Some provoked tears, some smiles, and some real laughter. Then, if a family member was present, he or she would walk to the altar escorted by one of the nurses' aides who cared for their relative. Together, they lit a memory candle. Often a spontaneous hug occurred at the altar.

One man's name brought forth this great story: "Remember when he first moved in? He was wearing an artificial leg he made himself out of a car door!"

After the service, as everyone enjoyed punch, coffee and goodies, more stories and memories were exchanged. The activities staff was beaming as the compliments flowed. "This sure made me feel better," said a nurses' aide.

Such observances can help all involved to complete their relationships with patients who have died and to celebrate those lives.

TODAY: Remember patients fondly.

Peeking into the day care center in the basement of the nursing facility, Bev watched her son playing with another boy. From the corner a toy came flying through the air, hitting her son in the leg. Her son then threw his toy, trying to hit his attacker.

As the day care staff settled the matter between the children, Bev went back to her duties considering what she had just seen.

"Am I really any different from my son?" she wondered. "Don't I want to strike back when something happens to me?"

Human beings do lead most of their lives in reaction. We're hit; we hit back. We're hurt; we hurt back. Such predictable behavior rarely makes us feel really powerful. More often we feel like victims—victims of each other, our bosses, the weather or whatever forces we feel controlled by.

To step out of this trap means to live no longer in reaction. The trick is to have a plan, a belief, a way of being that doesn't get rocked by every breeze and raindrop. That means that, no matter what cruel statement someone says to you or about you, you remain you. You continue to go about your day doing what you are paid to do.

A clever way to remember this healthy way of life is to write the word reaction on your piece of paper. Then, taking your pencil, erase the letter "c", and write another "c" at the beginning of the word. See? You're no longer living in reaction. You're living in creation. You create your day, your mood, your attitude. What freedom!

TODAY: Live in creation, not reaction.

Building a new nursing facility is an exciting project. What colors would you think are the nicest for bedrooms? Hallways? And how about the kinds of curtains? Everyone has their own opinions about what is right.

Walking through some new buildings, one wishes the architect had talked with the staff. What would they recommend for the kinds of windows? Floor coverings?

Sometimes what the staff and residents would prefer isn't glamorous enough for the marketing staff. After all, marketers want the place to look like a showcase, so families who feel guilty or sad about placing their relatives in a nursing facility will feel better.

Few of us will be able to help design a new institution. But that doesn't mean we cannot influence the interior decorating of the one we work in.

Staff at St. Joseph's Residential Care Home came in on their free time and painted all the trim in the old building. The bright, contrasting colors made every room look so lively. Someone found an old carved headboard in the basement, painted it, and hung it over the sliding window in the office. It looks like a gorgeous work of art!

In other homes, the staff has done stenciling to make the stark, bare walls more homey.

Two creative modifications to buildings have been reported by Nancy Mace, an Alzheimer's consultant. At the Minna Murra nursing home in Towomba, Australia, the staff installed brass door knobs for the patients to polish. At another unnamed facility, Ms. Mace said the staff so wanted to create a homelike environment rather than an institutional environment that they put an outhouse in the garden.

Can you top that?

TODAY: Cozy up your facility.

∞

June 9

How do you treat people who make mistakes? More importantly, how do you treat yourself?

Remember how relieved you were when, as a child, you made a mistake and your teacher was understanding? She might have even said, "That's okay. Making mistakes is how we learn."

The older we get, the more we kick ourselves when we make a mistake, believing that mistakes are always bad. Thomas Edison was once asked how he could possibly have invented so many successful projects—the electric light bulb and the phonograph, to name two.

"For every one good idea I have," the great inventor explained, "I have 500 bad ones." Thomas Edison saw failed ideas as simply part of the process. He didn't beat himself up or call himself a loser. He just kept on creating ideas.

Why not give yourself permission to make mistakes? We're not talking about mistakes born of sloppiness or neglect. But why not allow yourself the freedom of doing your best, trying some new ways, and not always hitting the bull's eye? It really is okay to make a mistake. Even geniuses do!

TODAY: Permit mistakes.

You see a lot of pain and suffering in your work. Part of your calling is to stand by your patients when that pain and suffering takes over. Sometimes, especially when the discomfort is physical, you can do more than be present. You actually can help get rid of the pain.

When the pain is emotional or spiritual, you face a tougher challenge. Loneliness is one diagnosis that staff can easily make. The cure is much more difficult.

LPN Bonnie Selberg (The Rotarian, July, 1992) writes of a wheelchair-bound patient who wished every day that his busy, successful son would visit:

> "Do you think he'll come today?" the old gentleman asks…Day after day, week after week, month after lonely month, the old-timer keeps this hopeless vigil, peering out the window of his small room, expecting to one day see his son walking up the sidewalk…How I wish I could say, "Yes! Today your son is coming!"…However, I am a nurse, and my profession demands honesty; so again this morning, I must gently tell him that I don't know if his son will come, but I will help him hope.

As this wise nurse points out, you can help your patients hope. Do not underestimate the power and value of this loving support. Hope is critical to our mental and physical well-being. Hope is that light in the darkness.

TODAY: Help your patients hope.

Eavesdropping on conversations in restaurants or at the bowling alley, it's often easy to hear meaningless chatter. People who are talking but not saying anything, staying with safe, worn words. Before we judge this kind of verbal idling, let's look at why we human beings are afraid to go into high gear and really say what we're thinking.

The key word is afraid. We fear the scary feelings and thoughts that might come up if we were to let our guard down. Nowhere is this frozen speech pattern more painfully present than when uncomfortable visitors come to call in the nursing facility.

James Campbell, in his delightful little book *What Do You Say? Learning to Listen for Grace in Nursing Homes and Other Care Settings,* writes:

> For all the concern about ecology, about preserving our resources, no resource is more carelessly wasted than the blessing of the old, withering in a silence of thoughtless relatives who visit and talk only of the weather, or clergy who come to preach with nothing to say yet preach anyway.

Instead of thinking that we have to do all the talking, Campbell suggests the key is not talking, but listening. He continues:

> I would not go with pity in my eyes and speak condescendingly about the weather. No, I would go passionately to listen. I would go to the nursing home seeking to be ministered to by these frail people who seemingly had nothing in life to live for. What do you say to people in care facilities, to shut-ins, to any person who by consensus has reached the point of being old? Nothing. If you really care about them, you go to listen, you go to be blessed.

TODAY: Listen, and be blessed.

"They didn't tie us up when we were held as prisoners of war," recalled a veteran of World War I, now living in a nursing facility. "I could never understand why they tied people here."

Looking back on what was once a standard nursing practice in nursing homes throughout the United States, many caregivers share the elderly gentleman's view.

Spurred on by a change in federal law, long term care facilities nationwide have been dramatically reducing the use of restraints, both chemical and physical. The results are gratifying. Residents are more lively and aware, and staff find themselves more satisfied at work, when people are not confined. Less time is spent on keeping people from doing things; more time is devoted to creatively responding to the real needs of residents. Staff can get back to the basics and take care of people.

Some staff are much less excited about freeing the patients, claiming the risks are too great. Employees worry about falls and wandering. Yet the question becomes: "Whose fear will govern you?" The resident's fear of being confined and tied, or the fears of the family, staff, and maybe the doctor's fear, all of whom claim it's for the patient's own good?

Maggie, a director of nursing, tells the story of the little lady who sat tied in a chair every day near the nurses' station. She had two pastimes: trying to untie her lap belt, and hitting everyone who walked by her. One day, after a particularly long struggle with the belt, the resident actually got it untied. She jumped up out of her chair, threw her hands in the air and shouted "Ta DA!"

"I saw how much it meant to her," Maggie said. "I decided we wouldn't tie her any more." Interestingly, once untied, the patient also stopped her second pastime of hitting. She now sits contentedly.

TODAY: Should you recommend someone be untied?

June was a lady. You could tell just by looking at her, just by being around her. There was a graciousness about her. She would always greet staff, strangers and visitors with the same lovely so-good-to-see-you smile.

Having lived her life by the etiquette book, it must have been hard for June to move into a nursing facility. So many of the daily acts of courtesy and civility are overlooked when people see each other day in, day out.

Jennifer, a certified nurses' aide, knew she was in the presence of someone of breeding and standing when she took care of June. In fact Jennifer sometimes felt she should call her Mrs. Rumley, not June. Not that June demanded that, or, in fact, demanded anything. She just commanded that kind of respect because she was so kind and appreciative herself.

Getting ten people out of bed and dressed in the morning was something Jennifer rushed through. There was little time for picking outfits or cleaning fingernails. A quick stroke with the hairbrush, maybe a dab of rouge, and whisk! On to the next patient. But Jennifer couldn't rush June Rumley. She was a lady who wanted to talk things over and wanted to hear how Jennifer and her family were. And she most certainly wanted her hair done one certain way. Given her pace, Jennifer simply could not devote the time to June's hairdo that was needed. She did her best and moved on.

But Jennifer wasn't just working to pay the bills. She worked because she loved the work. So, once a week, Jennifer stayed after work to visit and fix June's hair just the way she wanted it.

TODAY: What extra touch would bring a smile?

Have you heard this fairy tale?

It begins with your death. That's right. Get that scary thing over with, so you never have to dread it again. Then, move into a nursing home where the care is so good you are soon well enough to go home.

Once at home, you work hard in your chosen profession until it is time to retire and go to school. At school, you learn everything you want to know until you graduate and go home to your parents. At home, you play and have fun until you become a brand new, beloved baby. Then your life ends as a glimmer in someone's eye.

What a great, dreamy, way to live, to eliminate our fear of the end. Of course none can take a backwards journey. Instead we must face our fears head on, like it or not. As caregivers, you are called daily to help fearful and frail patients accept their journey.

The secret here is to remind patients that, yes, they will end up as a glimmer in someone's eye. Yours.

TODAY: Comfort frightened patients.

June 15

Working in healthcare, our moods essentially determine our effectiveness. We simply deliver a service and create relationships. When we are doing a good job, we see the results on our patients' faces. Folks are relaxed and hopeful around us. When we are doing a poor job, there is pain and tension present.

Weather reports are notorious for setting moods. Partly cloudy or partly sunny say the same thing, yet "partly sunny" fills me with hope; I hear "partly cloudy" and I start to droop.

Given the nature of patients' diagnoses, it is sometimes the biggest test of our day just to smile. Seeing or hearing all that pain and sorrow, depression and anger is almost more than we can bear.

But is it chicken or egg? That is, who causes whom to be bummed out? Try this experiment. Today look on the bright side every time you get a chance. The cup isn't half empty, it's half full. Your patient isn't an amputee, she has one good leg. You can't change them. But you can sure change you.

Treat your patients with this attitude and watch what comes back your way.

Write MOOD on a piece of paper and look in the mirror, holding it below your face. Now the word says DOOM. Don't let your face say DOOM too.

TODAY: Let the good moods roll.

The nursing home administrator was doing his best to create a feeling of team spirit at the facility. As a surprise at the staff picnic, he handed out free T-shirts with a mountain scene and the name of the nursing facility printed on them.

"I wouldn't be caught dead in one!" said an angry aide wearing jeans and a Bud Light T-shirt. How sad! She would advertise beer, but not promote the place she works, where she spends almost half of her waking hours?

Being angry at management and continuing to work there is just plain dumb. Nobody wins. The boss doesn't get respect; the staff can't have fun together; the residents really suffer. Just ask someone to comb your hair while she pretends she's mad. Doesn't feel very good, does it?

No work place is perfect, and nursing facilities can be tougher than many others. If you would rather not deal with people, get a job at the mill or the recycling center. Yes, you've got bills to pay, but nobody is forcing you to work as a caregiver. For everyone's sake, decide if you're in or out. If you're in, hang on for the ride. You're going to have a great time.

TODAY: Make sure you could wear a facility T-shirt proudly.

Hold out your hands. Are you giving or receiving?

If you answered "both!" you're right. Your busy, tired and probably chapped hands do plenty of giving and receiving all day long. What comfort they bring! While some psychologists talk about the value of living near relatives and the value of kinship, you know firsthand the value of "skinship"! A pat on the back, a reassuring squeeze at bedtime, a tap on the shoulder are all brought to you by hands.

Your devoted little hands do their best every day. They don't call in sick or stay in a bad mood, and they don't pretend they didn't hear what you asked them to do. They just get the job done.

Look at patients' hands. What kinds of stories do they tell? Notice the dairy farmer's big hands; they look like baseball gloves! Or see the grandma who has knit sweaters and mittens for almost eighty years. Notice the rings they still wear (sometimes arthritic knuckles have forced off all jewelry). Ask your patients to tell you about their rings. When did they get them? Where were they the day they received them? Who gave them?

Hands have plenty of stories to tell.

TODAY: Read some hands.

Statistics show that, nationally, the incidence of suicide in men over the age of seventy-five is high. We sometimes think suicide is the tragic accident of teenagers alone, but not so. According to the Center for Disease Control in Atlanta, the suicide rate among the elderly is nearly 8 percent higher than it is among people ages fifteen to twenty-four. Coping with loss of good health, independence, and family can be more than some people can bear.

For men who have found their identity through physical activity, being confined to a nursing facility bed or wheelchair may feel worse than death itself.

Physician-assisted suicide is not a new phenomenon, but widespread reporting about it is. For many years, compassionate doctors have listened to their patients' pleas to end their suffering and misery. Staff in hospitals and nursing facilities hear these pleas too—and are torn over what is the correct response.

In some instances staff have come upon a patient who has taken his or her life. No one can be prepared for such a moment. All facilities have protocols for handling these events.

If you have a patient who begins talking to you about suicide, report the conversation to your supervisor at once. No one expects you to provide mental health services to a troubled patient.

TODAY: Get your patients needed help.

On a cold winter day, a day most would say it was too cold to be outside, I drove by the public library. A crew of strong men was bringing a giant tree down onto the snowy lawn. As their arms wrapped around the huge trunk, I felt my heart sing the tree's joy. Here men, who weren't even alive when she was a young sapling, were carefully, lovingly taking care of her on her last day.

No amount of planning or investing or saving lots of money could have guaranteed to those who planted the elm that she would be laid to rest with tender care. The planters and the tree had to trust that the universe would provide, on the appointed day, the perfect team of people to do the job.

Caregivers in nursing facilities are just like that tree crew. Not around at the birth, they are called in at the end to ease the pain, to share the joy, to provide the regard and respect.

When my son was little, we were walking downtown. He had his new squirt gun and was learning the lesson about not pointing his pistol at living things. "Mom," he asked, gesturing to a hedge of cedar, "Is that a loving thing?"

Yes. A loving and a living thing, I told him, sharing the earth with us, deserving good treatment.

You are the caregivers tending to life's garden, to the mighty forests of old oak trees resting in your care.

TODAY: Tend loving and living things.

It's a hot afternoon, and nobody can get cool.

An ideal day to go out to the river and sit under the willow with a fishing pole!

Could this be the day you talk the activities staff into a spur-of-the-moment fishing trip?

Gloria was successful when she popped the idea on the activities department. "I've got plenty of poles at home; some are kinda old, but they can catch fish!" Gloria said.

The timing was perfect. Nothing was planned for the afternoon, so a group of five residents, wheelchairs and all, got into the van and headed off to buy some worms.

After two hours of fishing and plenty of story-telling, the creel was full with sunfish.

Back at the facility, the kitchen got into the spirit. Another group of residents volunteered to help clean the fish and make chowder.

That night the happy fishermen, the cooks, and the hungry bystanders enjoyed a special meal and some great stories about the one that got away.

TODAY: Hang up the Gone Fishin' sign.

Regret is a painful game. Playing the "if onlys" with yourself can be a cruel exercise with little positive outcome.

Marge was in her late fifties and had worked as an LPN for more than twenty-five years. She had planned to become an RN, but there was always some reason she couldn't go back to school. Her husband got sick and couldn't work; her daughter moved back home with two children; a favorite aunt needed lots of attention in her final years. Watching the new RNs come into the facility, making good money and having plenty of authority, was hard on Marge. At first she was angry at all the people in her family she had cared for instead of pursuing her education. Then, her anger shifted to herself. "I'm such a sap! Why did I let them use me?" she wondered.

Counselors who work with people in mourning explain the five stages of grief as denial, anger, bargaining, depression and acceptance. These stages apply to any experience of loss, be it a death or, in Marge's case, the loss of a dream. She bounced around the stages, sometimes feeling sad, other times pretending it didn't phase her.

The day Marge accepted her life and made peace with herself was the last day of her patient Russell's life. "I want you with me; I want to see your eyes last," he said hoarsely from his deathbed.

"I love you, Marge," Russell added. "I love you, too," Marge said. Russell then closed his eyes and died.

Reflecting on Russell's death, Marge said, "I wouldn't trade my life with anyone. I am so lucky." As the great writer Oliver Wendell Holmes wrote, "Every calling is great when greatly pursued."

TODAY: No regrets.

Some of us have chronic health problems—stomach upset, bad backs, headaches. We all have our weak spots, where stress and anxiety come to rest.

Articles about maintaining good health will often split the word disease, so it reads dis-ease. That is, our bodies are not at ease, the consequence being sickness.

Looking at your own recurring ailments, what can you see? Are you ignoring the messages your body is sending you about being uncomfortable, stressed out, hurting?

My friend Cindy tells me that she unknowingly keeps her shoulders hunched up until she causes herself a severe neck and shoulder ache. Why? "Because I'm trying to protect myself; I'm getting ready to defend myself; I'm trying to be perfect." Cindy is now learning to relax her shoulders and neck, and to be at ease.

In a dream one night, the words "healthy self" appeared floating in air. As I watched them they slid apart and then read "heal thyself."

We can go to plenty of doctors and emergency rooms and can get plenty of x-rays, prescriptions and even operations. But can we not do more with self-care, to "heal thyself"? Becoming aware of our own needs and limitations is a sign of true wisdom. Listen to what your body is telling you. See what you can figure out before you ask someone else to translate the messages.

TODAY: Heal thyself.

How many times do you enter a patient's room to be greeted by one or more complaints?

"The donuts were greasy this morning. My laundry came back all pink. No one has brought me my mail in two days."

It's hard sometimes not to blow your top. Wouldn't you like to recite some of your complaints to a captive ear?! At Eden Park Nursing Home in Rutland, the now retired administrator, Joan Fletcher, invented a simple and successful complaint system.

At the monthly resident council meeting, she asked for volunteers to help field facility complaints. "I need a patient who will listen to all the complaints about the kitchen and then come to me. I don't want my staff getting complaints every time they turn around—it is discouraging. The volunteer who takes this on must be willing to listen to all resident complaints about food."

Eva volunteered. Now, when a complaint about the dietary department is made, the resident is referred to Eva. Eva listens, writes it in her little notebook and saves it for a meeting with Mrs. Fletcher.

"They changed bakeries now," Eva said proudly. "I told them there were a lot of complaints about greasy donuts and they changed." The system works.

TODAY: Create a complaint system that works.

Tonight, at home, find some cardboard (a cereal box works well) and cut it up into small credit-card shaped pieces. (I trace a playing card.)

Tomorrow, in the break room, hand the cards out and tell your coworkers, "I want you to write three good things about how you do your job."

Guaranteed—everyone will look at you and say, "What?"

Just continue: "Please jot down three examples of the good job you do here. Like, 'I take time and do Miriam's nails' or 'I pitch in and help activities when they're short.' Write whatever little examples come to your mind, especially stuff that no one else has noticed or thanked you for."

At this point staff might act like they don't want to do this, but they do know what you mean. Be patient with them. They aren't used to complimenting themselves. When everyone is done (just a couple of minutes is plenty) tell them, "This is your personal credit card. Carry it in your wallet. Don't leave home without it. When you are feeling down, thinking that you aren't making any difference here, take it out and read it. Remind yourself of your worth. Give yourself some credit."

If you can convince them, it's fun to have everyone go around the room and read to each other what they wrote. Or just pass them around.

TODAY: Make personal credit cards.

One of my most powerful childhood memories was my Mom reading to me the book *I'll Be You and You Be Me* by Ruth Krauss.

As an adult I look at the vividness of this memory with a sense of mystery. Why did that moment and that book grab me so?

There are lots of funny little stories in this illustrated book, stories which prize imagination. Characters pretend and wonder about grand events and possibilities.

My favorite page, though, has always been the one with the big girl and the thin girl. It has five boxes, and this is what it says:

> She's wide and I'm thin—her hair's short and my hair's long—I hope I widen out as she grows narrowed and my hair should get shorter as hers gets long—we'd be like twins.

This page shaped my character. I see it everywhere. Can you see it in the Buddhist principle, "It is important to realize our sameness as human beings"? Or in these words from *The Magic of Conflict* by Thomas Crum?

> We begin to know the joy of service and to somehow sense that every time we add value to the lives of others, we are also adding value to our own. Ironically, giving becomes a self-serving act, as we find it impossible to distinguish where we end and where the outside world begins.

Can you see it in your nursing home? Can you see the sameness in your patients? Can you see it in yourself?

 TODAY: You be me, and I'll be you.

The old priest, long retired, sat in the wheelchair at the front door, greeting strangers as they came in. This station felt familiar to him. How many years had he waited at the door of another institution, the church, and welcomed strangers to his house of comfort?

No longer mentally alert or physically strong, Father Brevard still wore his clerical collar and garb. After all, he was still a priest.

Most of your patients don't have uniforms from their early years. The former bread truck driver no longer wears his blue shirt and pants. The old motel housekeeper isn't in her white pant suit. And the mailman turned in his uniform a long time ago.

It's almost too bad these folks are in civilian clothes now, because it makes it harder for you to know them. Without a strong work identity, many patients are not real people to us. Without seeing them in their home, we can't fully appreciate who they are.

My husband practiced medicine for almost twenty years and helped at more than 3,000 births. Only a small percentage of these babies were born at home, yet these are the births he remembers best. Why? Because they were so personal, with all the colors, smells and sights of a private home.

Without a home or a job, your patients may not appear as real people to you. Some facilities are asking families to bring in scrapbooks, so staff can see pictures of Mr. Jones when he was in his Army uniform or sitting strong and proud on his tractor. A few treasured items from home to decorate the patient's room can make a huge difference too. If the family members say "He doesn't even know where he is now; it wouldn't mean anything for him to have his army medals on the wall," tell them it would mean something to you.

TODAY: Take care of lifetimes, not just the end.

Laughter is the best medicine and just may be your best defense against insanity!

Pam Prue, an extraordinary activities staffer, lives this philosophy.

One of this lively lady's secrets to a joy-filled day is her costume closet. Big enough to hold a small meeting in (if it weren't so jammed), the closet is stuffed with outfits for every occasion. There's a gorilla suit, a nurse costume (large), clown clothes hanging beside stilts, squirting flowers and wacky wigs.

When the mood or the moment strikes her, Pam gets dressed. Patients never know what crazy garb Pam will appear in, which is half the fun of living at the facility.

One year, for her birthday, the staff all signed their names on a bright pair of boxer shorts. What a great gift for the costume lady!

On her next birthday, Pam approached a new staffer and said, "This was a great birthday, but I liked what I got last year even better."

The innocent newcomer went for Pam's bait. "What did you get last year?" she asked.

"These!" laughed Pam as she dropped her drawers and modeled her birthday boxers.

At some level, we all have a little Pam in us, begging to jump out. Encourage yourself today to do the goofy thing you've thought about for months. Sign someone's underwear!

TODAY: Be goofy.

"Behavior modification" is a popular way of treating problem children. The idea is simple enough—teachers reward good behavior and discourage bad behavior. After some time in such a classroom, difficult students are supposed to willingly modify their own behavior and improve.

In a nursing facility with patients who have problems, it is tempting to think behavior modification might be the answer. Another popular approach is called "reality therapy," where confused patients are consistently reminded, "No, Mrs. Frost. It is not 1935 and your daughter is not waiting for the bus. It is 1996 and you are in a nursing home."

Both methods are bad ideas in nursing facilities. We aren't dealing with children who need to learn the rules of society and be socialized. We are dealing with adults who no longer have the mental ability to understand the difference between good and bad behavior or between reality and fantasy.

In our situation the only behavior we can modify is our own. And the only reality important to the patient is his or her own.

In Japan, at the Sansuien facility, administrator Kentaro Ishi tells his staff that, while they can't always figure out what patients are thinking, that doesn't mean the patients should be forced to enter the staffs' reality. Sansuien staff, for example, make sure they relate to former corporate executives in an especially respectful way, asking questions and making comments that are suitable for the big boss.

In Vermont, the Building Bridges project promotes the same careful planning. Staff are encouraged to create activities and approaches that comfort the patients wherever they think they are. The retired nurse, now a patient, is given a huge stack of discarded files to shuffle through every morning. The former teacher has a desk and chalkboard for her use.

As long as no one is made fun of in the process, accepting the patient's view of the world is the kindest care we can provide. When we confirm their reality, it can bring comfort and peace.

TODAY: Modify your behavior.

Ever heard of the back door approach? Or a back-handed compliment?

When you practice these ways of being with people, it means that you indirectly make your point or give praise.

In a nursing facility, it is not tough to identify the nurses who don't belong there. The sour expressions, nasty comments and suspicious looks are instant identifiers. Such unhappy staff usually devote a great deal of their time to picking on others and finding fault. Not content to be miserable alone, they want everyone around them to suffer.

Unless you are in a management position, it can be awfully rugged dealing with such personalities. They seem to set you up and then catch you before you even notice what is happening.

Using the back door and slightly backhanded methods, though, you can have some influence.

Today, talk with other staff and set up a monthly staff-directed contest. Call it "Nurse of the Month" or "Employee of the Month," to be selected by the staff by secret ballot. Make a list of qualities you base your vote upon and (here's the backhanded part) make sure to choose qualities that are exactly the opposite of the grouch who has got your goat. Cheerful, sunny disposition, kind, helpful, team player—you get the picture.

Each month name one of the fine nurses or employees at your facility, make a little sign in her honor for the lobby, and even have someone make a cake for the break room. Of course, run the idea by your administrator. Tell him or her you want to recognize good staff rather than just complain about troublemakers.

After a couple of months, don't you think some of the negative staff will begin to wonder why they have never been honored?

TODAY: Use the back door.

Frank had been a bridge builder in the city of Boston in the 1930s. Later he built roads right through the White Mountains of New Hampshire. He was a man's man. Never married and never wanted to. His wardrobe consisted of work pants, work boots, plaid shirts and T-shirts.

Now his diabetes had claimed both legs and his once huge frame was propped up in a wheelchair. His voice was still pretty robust, and in fact someone was always complaining about how loud Frank was talking.

One day he asked a staff person to get him an application for a wild turkey hunting license. "The season's about to open, and I need my license," he said with a strong voice.

"Why do you need a license?" the young aide asked.

"I told you—the season is almost open!" Frank answered with impatience.

The aide went to the social worker, Barbara, and relayed Frank's message. "Thanks for telling me," the social worker said. "I always want to hear the special requests."

Down in Frank's room, Barbara told Frank that she heard he wanted a wild turkey hunting license. "Tell me about the turkey you've hunted, Frank," Barbara asked earnestly.

For the next thirty minutes, Frank told his wonderful hunting stories of the White Mountains before bulldozers had cut the roads. Why, Frank said proudly, he had kept a wild turkey hunting license in his wallet ever since they were first issued.

Realizing what having this license in his wallet meant to Frank, Barbara made the arrangements. Not much later, the license arrived in the mail.

Putting the license in its reserved spot in his wallet, Frank talked especially loud that day, showing it to all who had time to stop and listen.

TODAY: Keep traditions alive.

July

July 1

When your life is about taking care of sick people, it's amazing how much you can ignore your own illnesses.

A typical caregiver often wears a wrist brace or Ace bandage, has a bad cough, a chronic headache or other symptoms. Like the mythological wounded healer, the healthcare worker plugs along, putting one step in front of the other, ignoring her pain.

Few other people would so willingly go off to work on days when they felt so droopy. Such dedication speaks to the devotion that you have for your patients and your work.

The next time you find yourself heading off to work while ignoring an ailment, give yourself a little compliment. (If you're neglecting a serious problem, give yourself a kick in the pants and get to the doctor!)

Beyond this little act of self-praise, remember that you, even when you're sick or depressed, are a critical part of your patient's life. You are great. While you may feel like you're only half of your healthy self, you still are more than twice the average stranger walking through the facility. The way you care sets an example for all who know you. Thanks for hanging in there and being of service.

TODAY: See your dedication.

If your facility had a mascot, what would it be?

If you had a cheer, a motto or a secret handshake, what would it look like? Schools and sports teams have such traditions, even songs and anthems they sing about themselves. Churches have rituals and routines they observe regularly with a whole calendar of special days and seasons.

Look around you. What can you say about the team you serve on? Whom would you elect captain? Who would be the scorekeeper? The cheerleader?

Do you remember when the Atlanta Braves were in the World Series? The fans invented the "chop"—they brought their straight arms up and down imitating Indian tomahawks. Didn't someone just dream that up? You could do the same.

Watch the Boy Scouts or the Rotary Club open a meeting—plenty of little insider sayings and songs that bond the group together. I remember the first Rotary meeting I attended. A man announced he and his wife had a new baby. He passed cigars out to everyone present. Two minutes later everyone smoking a cigar was fined and the monies were paid to the club treasurer. The members loved this crazy practice, but I couldn't figure it out.

Why not invent some fun, specialized patterns and habits that your residents and staff can do together? How about a newsletter? Or buttons or baseball caps?

TODAY: Build your team.

As a child you learned almost everything you know by watching others. Sitting in your high chair or playpen, you saw your family go about their day-to-day business. At school, the teacher reinforced the family, reminding you about what was okay and not-okay behavior.

In trade industries, when someone wants to become a craftsman or artisan, they find an apprentice position. An apprentice is not just a follower, someone who imitates or copies the master. An apprentice is working to become a master, to use his or her gifts fully.

Remember your first day on the job? Who took time to show you, to teach you the facility's way of life? What did you learn from them? What did you choose to do differently?

Learning isn't just for children. As long as we are alive we are learning and growing. In the Christian church, different colored altar clothes decorate the church the whole year round, with white being reserved for holidays like Easter and Christmas. The two seasons of Ordinary Time, which follow Epiphany and Pentecost, are, however, marked by the color green, because it is ordinary to be green and growing. The normal state of a human being is to be growing.

To be ordinary, then, is to be constantly learning and teaching. Notice the teaching and learning your day includes.

TODAY: Teach and learn.

Independence is not something your patients know much about anymore. Few of them make such decisions as when to get out of bed, whom to associate with, what to do. Staff just hum along, making decisions for everyone. Not that staff are power-hungry or mean; it's just that it's easier to decide for others. With so much to remember and do, acts of convenience become very attractive.

Tressa Condon owns and operates, with her husband Phil, a small nursing home near the Canadian border.

"One day," Tressa said, "I was walking around the home and I realized we had patients who had not been out of the building, except to go to a doctor's appointment, in five years. I thought to myself, 'What makes us different from a prison?'"

That day Tressa decided that, at least one day a year, every person in the facility—staff and residents—would leave the building and the grounds and go somewhere.

When that summer day comes, a volunteer is found to answer the telephones, and the Condons and crew clear out.

One year they went to the beach. Another, to a state park. One year the residents won first prize in the Fourth of July parade. Some of the riders on the float were in bed, but they were there!

TODAY: Encourage independence.

Caregiving is surely not a "get rich quick scheme."

In our wealthy society, the poor are looked down upon as the lowest of the low.

Most of the patients in your facility are, probably, very poor—so poor they depend on government money to pay for their care. That money comes from taxes, and some of the taxes were paid by you. Kind of funny, huh?

If you've been in this work for awhile, you probably have accepted the low income as a way of life. You have settled for the other rewards that come with the territory.

Mother Teresa, the Catholic nun who founded the Missionaries of Mercy, is one of the most respected women on the planet. Having taken a lifetime vow of poverty, her life was about picking the dying poor off the streets and providing them with a clean, loving place to die. She refused all gifts and awards, and spent any money she was given on her patients.

In 1902, author, psychologist, and professor William James lectured in Scotland on the study of human nature:

> Among us English speaking peoples especially do the praises of poverty need once more to be boldly sung.... We despise anyone who elects to be poor in order to simplify and save his inner life. If he does not join the general scramble and pant with the moneymaking street, we deem him spiritless and lacking in ambition.

James continued, saying people had lost the ability to see the great value of choosing not to be rich. For him, being poor meant "paying our way by what we are or do and not by what we have."

You are paying your way through your daily acts of loving kindness. Like Mother Teresa, your pure life is about care.

TODAY: See how you pay your way.

For the past seven years, Gene Seese has wondered what it was like inside the small rural nursing home.

"I go to school right across the street," the thirteen-year-old said, "but this winter was the first time I ever went inside Stratton House." One of fourteen students participating in a service-learning project at Stratton House, Gene tends the pet fish and birds.

At Maple Lane nursing home, two pet llamas magnetize folks from far and wide. Calm, gentle creatures, they roam the fenced-in yard.

Does your nursing facility have friendly pets that make it comfortable for visitors to drop by?

Scruffy, the old Highland Terrier at Heaton House, is an excellent welcoming committee. And the two fat cats that live at Pleasant Manor Care Home are always looking for a lap and a handout. At the Gill Home, Seeing Eye dogs are trained right at the facility.

Residents also get a big kick out of pets. Literature produced by the AARP (the organization for retired people) declares that pets are good for your health. Summarizing the AARP position, it seems that people who care for another living being (such as a pet) always know that they themselves are needed. They know too that they must be reliable and plan for the future of the pet. Living for the future is the same as living in hope.

TODAY: Do you welcome pets?

Pet peeves are very personal, aren't they?

Nobody else finds these annoying little habits as grating as you do, darn it. If they did, maybe they wouldn't do them!

For years I have freaked out when, having finished my business on the toilet, I find there is no toilet paper on the roll. Gr-r-r-o-w-l.

At the time I make this discovery, I am long past the point of simply walking around the bathroom and looking into the cupboards. To do so would be to leave a trail! Complicating matters, this situation seems to occur most frequently in other people's offices or homes, where I don't know where the toilet paper is kept. Double g-r-r-o-w-l.

Around 1984, after a particularly aggravating experience of the N.P.P. (No Paper Phenomenon), I found myself back at my desk, writing a bitter poem about inconsiderate people who don't replace the empty roll (I think I called it an Ode. I was in a nasty mood.)

Quite suddenly, while writing, I realized my pet peeve had gained too much power. A poem? On toilet paper? I was out of control and it was time to transform this problem, I thought.

Drastic moods call for drastic measures. I decided that, from that moment forward, every empty roll I came upon would be a sign of good luck. The more empty rolls, the more good fortune would roll my way.

Call it crazy, but it has worked so well that I now thank my family for leaving me empty rolls! And instead of anger this new reaction has generated quite a few laughs.

A few summers ago, aboard a large ferry boat, my son came running out of the men's bathroom. Looking down from the upper deck into the crowd of tourists, he yelled "Mom! You're going to love the men's bathroom!" The crowd became silent, heads whipped around to see this kinky mom. My son continued in a loud voice, "There's no toilet paper!"

I'm sure those folks will take that puzzling incident to their graves.

TODAY: Transform your pet peeve.

I knew our eyesight fails as we age, but Lorraine, an RN, was the one who taught me how colors begin to fade and look washed out to old eyes.

An administrator of a community facility she helped design and build, Lorraine was always receiving donations from families. Often mentioned in a resident's will, her home regularly accepted gifts of cash and goods.

One year Mr. Lahey, an artist who had been a patient, died and left his entire collection of hundreds of oil paintings to the home. Lorraine converted her facility's halls into an art gallery and hung dozens of lovely landscapes throughout the building.

Looking at these paintings day after day, Lorraine discovered something about Mr. Lahey. His early art had vibrant and varied colors, but the older the artist got, the more he painted with predominantly muted shades of green and yellow. "His eyes were changing," Lorraine explained. "He couldn't see colors anymore; everything looked yellowish to him."

Think of this need for bright primary colors when you're picking out clothes for patients. If you can, make sure you dress in brilliant colors too.

TODAY: Add a splash of color.

Look around you. Saints walk among you in those wide, shiny halls.

I met Dee Dee one hot summer's night while visiting the nursing home where she worked as a certified nurses' aide. Normally a night aide had twelve people to get ready for bed. Tonight, because someone hadn't shown up for work, Dee Dee was responsible for sixteen patients.

Efficiently helping her patient from the wheelchair to the bed, Dee Dee looked over at me, a visitor in the room. "I know I probably don't look like I know what I'm doing," she said. I had noticed she had asked the patient a few things about what he needed before bed, but figured she was just being thorough.

"You see," she continued, "I don't usually work nights."

"Oh," I nodded. "Why are you working tonight?"

"Well, I got married today, but they called and said they only had two aides tonight and begged me to come in," she answered shyly.

"You got married today and you came to work tonight?" I said in shock.

"Yes. I just couldn't let the girls down. I knew two of them would have to take care of forty-eight patients. With me here, there are three to do the work," Dee Dee said.

We talked about how her husband had agreed to wait until tomorrow to go on their little honeymoon camping trip.

Dee Dee finished and went on to the next room. I sat, stunned, having seen selflessness as never before.

TODAY: See saints.

The story is told that Ivory soap, the only soap that floats, was invented quite by accident. In fact the inventor was at first fired by the soap company.

It seems a young man at the Ivory plant was supposed to switch the soapy soup from one tank to another. Instead he dozed, and the liquid soap was whipped much longer before it went down the line to be formed into bars. When his supervisor found him asleep at the button, he was dismissed.

Weeks later, when that batch of Ivory hit the stores, consumers started to notice their soap floated in the tub! Letters poured in to the company praising this convenient improvement. The baffled managers couldn't figure out what had happened. Following a detailed investigation, the company determined the extra stirring and whipping had pumped a lot more air into the mix. The air bubbles made the bars float!

At an old hospital-turned-nursing home, the new mother on staff had asked for any donations of baby clothes. "This is my first, and I'm starting from scratch," she said. Her coworkers came through, bringing little play suits and frilly dresses to work, putting them in a box by the coffee machine.

One day a wandering patient with Alzheimer's came upon the box. She picked up a pink, lacy frock and squealed with delight! She then removed a pale blue sweater, sat down and repeatedly folded and unfolded it.

From this accidental moment, the staff learned how many patients with dementia enjoy handling baby clothes. Now, a big box of "play clothes" is always

available in the activities room for patients to touch
and appreciate.

TODAY: Look for good fortune accidents.

Plenty of workshops and in-service training sessions are held every year on "standard precautions," those procedures followed to avoid the spread of communicable diseases. With the AIDS epidemic and the risk of hepatitis B always present, healthcare workers need to be rigorous in practicing infection control.

In the early 1990s, New England hospitals were hit by MRSA (methicillin-resistant staphylococcus aureus), a virulent staff infection that defies antibiotics.

Perhaps even more threatening to the well-being of a nursing facility is another kind of staff infection, one that poisons all it comes in contact with and spreads by word of mouth. Which staff infection is that? The bad attitude.

Surely you know the symptoms: difficulty smiling, heavy whispering, inability to pitch in and improve a situation.

While there is no known vaccine, such staff infections can be prevented. Stay strong. Resist the temptation to tear down and hurt others. Believe in your own inherent goodness and the goodness of others. Be healthy!

TODAY: Fight staff infections.

Newspapers are full of little articles underlining the ironies of life. Did you see the story of the Mt. Pleasant, NY, driver who was so angry at another driver who passed him on the highway? Seems the angry driver caught up with the passing car and drove beside him, swearing, honking and shaking his fist. This tirade went on until he lost control of his vehicle, rolled the car and died instantly.

Then there was the young man in Lincoln, Nebraska, who stole a checkbook and some identification. He went to a nearby bank to cash a check and presented his ID card, claiming he was Tim Holt. The problem was that the bank teller was the real Tim Holt, and the stolen ID was his!

As the saying goes, what goes around comes around. Life usually doesn't present us with such immediate returns. Few of us commit a mean, selfish or illegal act and get feedback so instantly. My fifth grade teacher, Alice E. McClay, said "Turnabout is fair play."

What are you dishing out? Is there any mystery about why you're getting what you get?

TODAY: Give what you want to get.

Ann Keenan first taught me about the importance of talking to people in a coma.

As a lifelong nurse, Ann had worked both in hospitals and nursing facilities. One of her patients was an elderly man in a coma. With no awareness of his surroundings, the man seemed as though he should die. Yet he hung on for no apparent reason.

Once a week the man's grown daughter would ride the bus from a neighboring town to sit at the foot of her father's bed. This habit intrigued Ann, as the woman never spoke to her father, and he didn't seem aware of her visit.

One night Ann said to the daughter, "I'm so curious about why you visit." The woman explained that her father had walked out on the family when she was a tiny child and that she had no memories of him. Quite by accident she had learned her father was a patient in the facility and had decided to visit.

"I wanted to experience being with my dad even if he doesn't know I'm here," the daughter said.

"Have you forgiven your father for walking out?"

"Oh, yes," the daughter said. "My mother remarried."

The nurse then looked at the young woman and said, "Would you go back in the room and tell your father you love him and that you forgive him?"

Without much hesitation, the daughter did just that. A few hours later the father died peacefully in his coma.

We can't begin to understand what people hear and don't hear in a coma. The lesson here, as Ann taught it, is that we need to talk with coma patients the same way we talk to the alert. In this case, a father needed permission to die.

TODAY: Talk to coma patients.

When I took my son's Cub Scout troop to a nursing facility one Christmas season, I was not prepared for how the young boys would visit.

Elliot, my son, has grown up around nursing facilities and their patients and is incredibly at ease and natural in the presence of frail old people. When he was just four years old, we visited a community care home where an old man sat in the hallway in his wheelchair motionless. The nurse told me he was "unreachable, in his own world."

Leaving Elliot in the big open hallway to push his matchbox car, I went into a nearby room to visit with another patient. Suddenly I heard a wild hooting from the hallway.

The "unreachable patient" was kicking the toy car to Elliot, and Elliot would rocket it back. Each trip produced a hoot from the elderly man, even a smile.

The other boys in Elliot's troop hadn't had this early experience, so they rode the railing in the hallway that Christmas time, clearly uncomfortable about visiting the old and infirm.

Bringing your children to work can be mighty important, more important than you may imagine. Not only does it perk up the patients and reconnect them with the wonderful world, but these interactions will open your children up to a lifetime of relating to old age. Kids will not be afraid of the old or of getting old. The simple act of bringing your kids into contact with your patients is one giant step for humankind.

 TODAY: Bring your kids to work.

July 15

One of the challenges of caring for people with very limited abilities is helping them be useful. Our society doesn't prize the disabled or elderly. Your job is about ignoring that prejudice and finding meaningful projects for patients.

At Crescent Manor in Bennington, many of the patients have done some sewing in their lives. While eyesight is failing and hands may be arthritic, uncomplicated crafts are still possible.

When the activities director heard that state social workers needed some teddy bears for abused and neglected children in state custody, a brilliant idea was born. Working with a simple pattern, the Crescent Manor residents make teddy bears for the needy children. The cuddly, cheerful bears are full of love and desperately needed.

Many such opportunities are available for alert residents to continue to participate in the life of the wider community. An enterprising group of women has created ABC or Aids Baby Comforters. This volunteer effort solicits handmade comforters for babies born with the deadly disease AIDS. (Contact Marie Davis, RR 1, Box 1505, Arlington, VT 05250 or the ABC Project nearest you.)

TODAY: Connect patients with projects.

The Bible is full of lessons about how to lead our lives. The story of Mary and Martha is well known. It tells the tale of how two sisters act when Jesus is visiting. Martha is super busy, cooking and cleaning and working in the house. Mary sits and spends time with Jesus, which makes Martha really mad. Martha complains to Jesus, and Jesus tells Martha to lay off, saying Mary made the right choice.

Most people interpret this parable to mean that being with people is more important than doing the housework. Your patients would probably agree. Walking through the halls at night, visitors will see the nurses all clustered around the medication cart. The patients are in beds, waiting for a visit.

Codependent No More is Melody Beattie's twenty-two pages of wise words. The subtitle of this stunning book, *How To Stop Controlling Others and Start Caring For Yourself,* is an invitation to many of us. Ms. Beattie interprets the Mary and Martha story this way:

> There's a message here about taking responsibility for our choices, doing what we want to be doing and realizing how we become angry when we don't. Maybe Mary's choice was right because she acted as she wanted to. Jesus helped many people, but He was honest and straightforward about it. He didn't persecute people after He helped them. And He asked them what they wanted from Him. Sometimes He asked why, too. He held people responsible for their behavior.

Take some time and look into your own caregiving patterns and behavior. Where do you go too far, crossing the line from the Land of Satisfaction to the Land of Resentment? How can you let more of the Mary out in you?

TODAY: Okay, Martha, cool your jets!

A frantic telephone call from a frantic relative of a nursing facility patient one Saturday morning: "They are trying to kill my mother!" she cried.

It seems her mother, a very ill patient, needed to be hospitalized for pneumonia. The mother didn't want to go to the hospital or take any medicine. In health-care lingo, she was "refusing treatment." Following doctor's orders, the nursing home staff called the woman's family.

"What should we do? Should we grant your mother's wishes and keep her here, out of the hospital and comfortable?"

The middle-aged daughter freaked out. To her, not doing everything medically possible to treat her mother, regardless of her mother's wishes, was "like murder!"

Looking into the situation, I learned the mom had been biting staff and refusing food for some time. The daughter told me she and her father had decided to "keep mom alive for as long as we can whatever it takes."

There you have it. Responding to their own needs and not necessarily to what their sick loved-one wanted or needed, the family was mad at the care-givers. Caught in the middle, the nursing facility was cast as the bad guy.

As you know, this kind of case is not that unusual. Unable or unready to deal with the loss of a mother or wife, the relatives panic and deny reality. Your job is to take care of your patient, being sensitive to the emotional state of the family. Not a simple assignment.

TODAY: Help families see reality.

When an idea is a great idea, the benefits are unbelievable.

Take the plant project at the Helen Porter Nursing Center in Middlebury. First the idea was simply to have interested patients, in late winter, plant seeds in indoor pots. The tiny plants would be moved to an outdoor garden when all fear of frost had past.

In late summer someone suggested other interested residents might like to press the flowers and make stationery, lamp shades and other gifts.

After that, when it was harvest time, someone suggested making relishes and chutneys with the green tomatoes and other vegetables.

With all these goodies, it was a logical step to have a craft and food sale with still other interested residents serving as salesmen and women.

TODAY: Have a great idea.

Kathy and her sister Judy have worked at the Manor for so long that it probably should be called Kathy and Judy's Manor. Having worked their way up the staff ladder, they are now administrator and director of nursing.

Don't tell these ladies that something is not possible. "Not possible" seems to be a code phrase that triggers their unconscious into hearing a "no problem" approach.

Take the summer the two women decided what the residents really needed was a nice deck off the back of the building. By the time they finished describing this addition, everyone could picture the deck and all the fun it would permit.

But the out-of-state owner told Kathy and Judy that, with a tight budget, the deck was "not possible."

But don't worry. After all, Kathy and Judy didn't. Remember, when others hear "not possible," they hear "no problem." The two simply kicked into their overdrive gear and organized bake sales, lawn sales, raffles—you name it. By the end of summer, the deck was done and all paid for by donations and fundraisers.

TODAY: Hear "no problem."

Creativity is such a wonderful commodity in a nursing facility.

Years ago the Alcoa Company, an aluminum processor, produced a film called *Why Man Creates.* In it the filmmaker tackles the question of what being creative is and where creativity comes from. In essence the film concludes that we create to express our identity, to say "I am." Creativity, it postulates, "is seeing one thing and calling it another."

That's why half-gallon milk cartons in some facilities become busy boxes. Staff brainstorm about activity themes such as fishing, sewing, cooking, baking, makeup and hair care. Then donations of items associated with these themes are collected and put in a busy box. When a confused resident is agitated, staff grab one of the busy boxes and see if the items will interest the resident for a few minutes.

Designing clever projects doesn't have to cost a lot of money or require a lot of time. Shoestring budgets, in fact, often produce the most fun. Spelling bees are always successful, especially if you add a little spice, as did the nursing facility that challenged the minor league baseball team to a spell-down. (Most of the players were foreign, and the patients did incredibly well!) Or the time the Governor was invited to the current events discussion group.

Giving a little twist to the predictable is just the creative touch your patients will love. And work is less like work when creativity is in action.

TODAY: See one thing and call it another.

One aspect of quality health care is tough to understand: the illusive quality of quality itself! Supervisors feel obligated to emphasize the importance of quality, particularly if it's absent. And staff like to think they don't need to be told; of course we know what quality care looks like!

Still, there must be specific standards of care that patients and their families can count on.

The old Chinese koan asks the question, "If a tree falls in the forest when no one is there, does it make a sound?"

Customized to the care setting, the koan might read, "Is quality care provided even if no one is watching?" When the supervisor isn't present, the visitors have gone home and the state inspectors aren't around, does that confused patient get the same quality TLC?

A minister once preached a sermon on the importance of all people being honest in all of their dealings with others. He pressed his congregation to look deep into their lives and root out all dishonest practices.

The next day he rode a city bus downtown.

Having paid his fare and found a seat, he walked back up to the driver. "Excuse me, driver, but you gave me $1 too much in change."

"I know," said the driver, keeping his eyes on the road.

"Why?" asked the minister.

"I was at your church yesterday. I just wanted to see if you really practice what you preach," the driver answered.

What can be said about the quality of care you provide behind closed doors? Does your performance vary, depending on who's present?

TODAY: Quality is quality is quality.

Suicides and homicides in the homes of the rich and famous always seem to intrigue us. How could a person who has seemingly everything be that unhappy?

As human beings, we are constantly trying to figure out if, indeed, you can tell a book by its cover. Are pretty people really better? Can money buy happiness?

When families shop for nursing facilities, this question about appearances takes on great weight. Does the fancy foyer with the six-foot palm plants mean mom or dad will get terrific attention and care? What about the lovely wallpaper? Does that mean patients don't get sad and blue?

Certainly pleasant surroundings do influence how human beings feel. Just ask anyone who has spent time in prison. The environment does make a difference. But how much?

I remember talking with the staff of a truly old building, a nursing facility that, in its prime, had been a striking Victorian mansion. Today it was like a run-down old bag lady in need of money and care.

"When families come to check us out, they always talk about how old our linoleum looks and the dark, narrow hallways," the staff lamented. "They talk about how the other home in town is so bright and cheery."

Hearing this frustration I felt like the mother whose daughter says she wants to have a nice bike like the rich girl next door. "It isn't fair," she agreed. "I wish I could change things."

If you are working in a facility that is no showboat, remind each other that looks are only a small part of the story. More important than the set and the props are the actors and their lines. When caregivers are stars, no amount of expensive interior decoration can compare.

TODAY: Let your light shine.

Every society has its own way of meeting the needs of the vulnerable. In this country, the responsibility for the frail among us has continued to shift from the family to government. Once people took care of old relatives at home. Now, with women working, children and aging parents are sent to day care. Many of the elderly end up in nursing facilities.

Few of us are prepared to pay our way in an institution. No matter how frugal we've been, it's doubtful we have $35,000 in the bank for a year of nursing facility care. Without means, needy old folks end up going onto welfare. Welfare, for most Americans, is a dreaded system. Your patients probably worked long and hard all their lives, never depending on a handout or the government dole. To end up poor and sick is not part of anyone's plan.

In England a special association exists to provide monies for similarly afflicted elders. The organization, known by the wonderful name Distressed Gentlefolks' Aid Association, caters to members of grand families down on their luck.

Isn't that name beautiful? It is so dignified and respectful! It hardly clangs of "public assistance" or "welfare." Aiding distressed gentlefolks sounds so delicate.

Many of the people you care for don't know they are totally dependent on the government to pay the bills. Such an announcement would crush their pride, their sense of self-worth. You don't deal with the billing; you can remain pure and neutral in the delivery of care. Everybody is equally treated under your hands. In fact you can simply see yourself as aiding distressed gentlefolks who are down on their luck. That's a position any of us can find ourselves in.

TODAY: Aid distressed gentlefolk.

Author John Steinbeck saw humanity in very black and white terms. He claimed there were two kinds of people in the world—those who would go out of their way to avoid hitting a turtle crossing the road and those who would go out of their way to hit that turtle.

Quite an image, huh? Setting aside the debate about whether these two categories actually cover all people, let's consider the concept.

Look around the building. Among the staff, are there any turtle killers? Aren't they the very individuals you have trouble with, the very employees you wish worked elsewhere?

And how about the residents? Are there any turtle killers in their ranks? Don't you have similar thoughts about them? Human beings who don't appreciate and value life are difficult to be around.

As a caregiver, you are called to be evenhanded with all in your charge. But does that mean you work side-by-side with coworkers who are known for their insensitivity, nastiness, even cruelty? What is your responsibility as a staff member?

While we all have our own work styles, it seems we owe it to our patients, at the very least, not to ignore turtle killers in our midst. These kinds of people don't belong in the caregiver role. They belong in jobs with inanimate objects like machines and paper. We can try as hard as we can to work with mean-spirited coworkers, but there comes a point when they need to move on. As an administrator once told me, "They aren't bad people. They just want to play basketball and we're about baseball. They are interested in a different game, not the one we are playing here."

TODAY: Talk to your supervisor about turtle killers in your midst.

∞

Nelda Samarel, a professor at William Patterson College, wrote a book in 1991 entitled *Caring for Life and Death*. Her book reported on the results of a study she conducted exploring how nurses treat two different types of patients at the same time—the terminally ill and those who are expected to recover.

Ms. Samarel's study identified two factors that influenced the way nurses care for their patients. "One, the patient's level of consciousness (that is, whether or not the patient is responsive), and, two, the 'busyness,' or amount of work required by each nurse on any given day."

No surprises here, right? Caregivers in nursing facilities are well aware of these two factors. When someone doesn't say "thank you," or for that matter say anything at all, it can be hard to stay tuned in and interested in them as a caregiver. We all need feedback. Look how long strangers will talk to a baby in a restaurant or store, hoping to elicit one of those precious baby smiles.

And that darn "busyness" Ms. Samarel refers to—what a pain! For nurses and, increasingly, nurses' aides, we're talking about paperwork here—"paper compliance" in regulatory terms. Marking down who got what medicine and when, and who refused what medicine and when. Such tedious accountability can sure take the joy out of the job. But Ms. Samarel also found that:

> Nurses who develop a philosophy of death, participate in regular support groups and continuing education programs, and have time to

enact and reflect upon their caring behaviors are best able to make the transition between different types of patients and to give the care that is required of them.

Some surprises here, right? Did you know how important it is that you develop a personal philosophy of death? And a support group where you can talk about the job? Did you realize how valuable ongoing training is to your performance? And how you need to make time to notice what you are doing on the job?

These insights are 100 percent wisdom. Share them with your employers today. See what you can set up to meet your needs and to assure your success in this career.

TODAY: Begin a support group.

Annual inspections by the state can send chills down even the most secure administrator's spine. Nobody looks forward to these mandatory visits.

In most states, such yearly reviews are unannounced, the government believing that the surprise element catches a facility in a more typical day. From the staff's standpoint, the unexpected nature of the inspection produces huge amounts of tension. Nobody likes company to arrive unexpectedly.

The common practice is for a team of state nurses to tour the facility over a certain period of days studying every aspect of the operation. Nothing escapes their eyes, be it the temperature of the bath water or how quickly residents are fed their meals.

Following the inspection, an exit interview is held with key staff. At this time the state team shares the basics of their findings, promising a written report to follow. Facility staff can challenge or respond to the team's findings.

I often wonder what it must be like to serve on one of these inspection teams. Clearly, no one welcomes your presence. The job must be fairly thankless.

From the facility's standpoint, these licensure-renewal visits can be quite demoralizing. Linden Lodge was cited for failure to administer drugs properly. Sounds pretty serious, until you hear that it means a nurse crushed a pill for a patient who had trouble swallowing, but without a doctor's order. And Berlin Health and Rehabilitation Center was cited for not meeting the sanitary standards for food handling—by leaving a scoop in the oatmeal bin.

Such deficiencies don't accurately tell the story of care at these nursing facilities. Yes, objective inspections are valuable, as they give the staff another perspective. No, we cannot rely upon these state reports as complete pictures of a home's performance. An inspection is merely a snapshot in time.

TODAY: Don't get discouraged by the inspectors.

As a professional caregiver, you should read Dr. Bernie Siegel's books. One of the truly gifted healthcare authors of this century, Bernie Siegel is a Yale surgeon who writes about the power of love and positive thinking in our healing.

In his bestseller *Love, Medicine and Miracles,* Bernie wonders why God doesn't give humans a reset button like the one installed on a garbage disposal. He writes:

> God answered, "I did give you a reset button, Bernie. It's called pain and suffering. It is only through pain that we change. It can be difficult to see our loved ones hurting but not changing. Our job is to love them. It is their pain that changes them, not our sermon."

Sometimes, when the pain our patients are suffering is so obviously self-inflicted, we're tempted to give a little lecture or mini-sermon. Mrs. Tenney's back and knees hurt. Why wouldn't they? She is almost 150 pounds overweight! No wonder her body can't take the load. Or what about the diabetic who insists on smoking, seated in her wheelchair after a leg amputation?

Bernie Siegel reminds us to avoid jumping up on our soapbox and preaching about all the things patients are doing wrong and what bad people they are. Our call is not about producing quick fixes. It is about love—loving people in their present condition, with no strings attached. Let them reach the point of transforming pain into change.

TODAY: No preaching, just loving.

He was a retired bachelor dairy farmer. Selling his farm to a big city developer for housing lots, Fred had made a tremendous amount of money. With no family, he had put his money in the bank and moved into a small retirement home.

Fred had seen me, the young state worker in the building, visiting other residents. He informed the staff that, he, too, needed an appointment with the state worker. "I want to talk to her about my bank books," he explained.

Not much later I paid a visit. Fred launched into his tale, something about being worried about whom to will his money to. "You know," he offered, "the right woman could inherit a fortune if she were to marry me now."

Every time I would make a suggestion, Fred would say, "I can't hear you." This problem would bring me a little closer to Fred, until I was finally one inch from his ear, speaking loudly. Fred still said he couldn't hear what I had to say.

Meanwhile, two employees of the home were walking by Fred's door. "Did you bring Fred his laxative this morning?" one whispered to the other.

"Yes she did! Now go away and don't disturb me and my lady friend!" Fred yelled out the door. Amazed at his improved hearing, I pulled away from Fred, who had managed to have one arm around my waist.

Laughing later with my boss, I realized I had learned a lesson that day—never underestimate the vitality of a man!

TODAY: Watch for winks!

Few patients seem like they belong in a nursing facility. Some appear more able to adjust than others. The younger the person, the harder it can be to live in an institution.

The family of a younger patient often struggles with this. How many mothers anticipate seeing their beloved eighteen-year-old son, head injured in a motorcycle accident, drooling in a wheelchair?

Marcia's situation was just that. Five years earlier her son Evan survived a serious crash that left him with the mental ability of a child three months old. Once self-sufficient and stubborn, Evan now needed everything done for him, from feeding to diapering.

A motel housekeeper, Marcia would try to visit Evan every day on her way to or from work. She wanted to check on her boy, to touch him.

One night she arrived after dinner and began to wash Evan for bed. On the night stand was a bottle of lotion with a sticker that read, "Staff Only. Not the Mother."

Telling a friend later about this sticker, Marcia cried: "I have so little with my son, why would they want to take this away from me?"

It seems some nurses didn't like what they saw as Marcia's interference. Not feeling Marcia's pain, they caused her more.

TODAY: Feel families' pain.

In tough economic times, salesmen and women have to be pretty creative to earn money. For a shoe salesman in Woodstock named Herbert, creativity came naturally.

One day at a Rotary luncheon, he heard a talk by the local nursing facility administrator. Approaching her after the meal, he made this proposal: "What if I drop by your place and see if anyone needs new shoes? I bet it isn't easy to come down to my store, so let me bring my store to you!"

The administrator was delighted, and invited Herbert to come by with a sample of his more comfortable shoes.

One night after work, Herbert dropped over with his shoes and his smile, but the evening wasn't anything like what he expected. "I couldn't believe how great I felt being there," he recalled later. "They were such lovely and interesting women. And they were so happy I came over; they treated me like a king!"

From that moment forward, Herbert made a decision to visit the home every Sunday morning. "I don't go to church," he said. "I come up and visit, and I feel really great when I go home."

TODAY: Invite some salespeople over.

Diets. Nobody likes them, and almost everyone is on one.

In nursing facilities, mealtime is an exciting time. Yet most residents are on restricted diets with purees, no salt, no sugar, no fat and, unfortunately, no taste.

At the Vernon Green Nursing Home, the staff decided such boring, bland diets were not at all appealing. "We like a treat and a sweet every so often; why shouldn't the residents?" said the administrator, Larry.

Working with the staff dietitian, the facility created a Dining with Dignity program, a no-restrictions menu. A pastry chef who specialized in butter-rich baked goods was hired. Cream, salt and other previously forbidden ingredients were added to recipes.

Of course patients with doctor's orders for reduced calories or other restrictions continue to eat the old way. But unless they are under restrictions, the residents of Vernon Green are enjoying culinary bliss.

"What does it matter if they gain a few pounds or have high cholesterol?" Larry asked. "Their average age is eighty-five. They can't live forever; why not make these remaining years delicious ones?"

TODAY: Talk about an expanded menu.

August

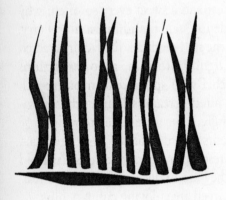

Late one Sunday night, I was driving in upstate New York, cruising the radio for an interesting program. Quite suddenly a frightened woman's voice came through the speaker: "We are really worried, doctor, about her quality of life. She doesn't eat much, is listless and some days sleeps twenty-three hours. The whole family wonders what we should do."

Wow! A show dealing with the final days and a family being forthright enough to confront the issues responsibly. I listened some more.

"Sometimes she has no control of her bladder; we have to wipe up a lot, doctor," the voice continued.

The doctor's response startled me, and then I caught on. The show was a pet show. The doctor was a veterinarian.

In our culture we're more able to talk about the difficult decisions surrounding aging pets than aging parents and grandparents.

Have you ever been in the room of a dying patient when nervous visitors arrived? Once such an awkward visitor walked in and saw the urine bag beside the bed. She blurted out to the dying patient, "My your urine is looking wonderful today!"

For all of us, even if we are blessed enough to live a long life, the end does come. While it is painful and awkward and sad, it is, above all, natural. Help others see this.

TODAY: Normalize death.

I heard recently of an archaeological dig that unearthed a human skeleton believed to be 60,000 years old. What was truly remarkable about the find was that the man had broken legs long before his death and thus lived while unable to walk.

The archaeologists and anthropologists studying the find cite these remains as empirical evidence of the beginnings of civilization. To survive, this disabled man had to have someone helping him, someone bringing him food and water and protecting him against harm.

Ultimately the true measure of a civilization, a society, is how people treat one another, how they care for themselves and others, well beyond mere survival.

Thousands of years from now, when a group of 50th century sociologists is studying the US culture at the turn of the 20th century, it will no doubt be intrigued by nursing facility CNAs.

Who were these saints who could have gotten a job doing almost anything else and earned more money? Who were these devoted souls who tended to the broken, ill and abandoned?

You are part of a great long chain of selfless caregivers who have made time for others.

TODAY: Acknowledge yourself.

Mr. Gannett was a true gentleman, obviously of fine stock.

Certainly he had a first name, but no one thought of using it. In his tie and sport coat, Mr. Gannett hadn't been called anything but Mr. Gannett since childhood, except by his wife. And she called him "Ganny."

Still dressed for success (he had been an investment banker) Mr. Gannett was no longer aware of his surroundings. He had a dementia diagnosis or was, as some would joke, "going head first."

Committed to Mr. Gannett's peace of mind, the nursing facility staff went to great lengths to keep a regular, predictable routine. The more they could maintain a feeling of the familiar for their patient, the less agitated he became.

Mornings were still difficult though. Mr. Gannett had accepted the fact that others were washing and dressing him. Toileting had been a real adventure. Finally someone figured out that giving Mr. Gannett his address book, or any book, preoccupied him, and they were able to get him on and off the toilet with relative ease.

But after he was fixed up for the day and had eaten breakfast (toast, tomato juice, hard-boiled egg and coffee), Mr. Gannett would become anxious and fidgety.

One day, when talking with his daughter, the nursing facility stumbled on an idea. Mr. Gannett needed his New York Times! "He read the Times every morning!" his daughter said with certainty.

Though Mr. Gannett could no longer read, a few copies of the Times were purchased and kept at the nurses' station. Every day a paper was brought in and placed in Mr. Gannett's lap. He became as calm as a kitten. The paper was returned to the nurses' station later in the day, then recycled back to Mr. Gannett the next morning. When it got too tattered, another was purchased, and always the New York Times and no substitute.

TODAY: Find the familiar and use it.

What do your patients need? What are you able to provide?

Libraries and bookstores have shelves full of books tackling the question of what do men and women need. Entire college degrees are wrapped up in the answers to this question.

Consider these eight points from an anonymous author:

1. The need for love and affection.
2. The need for security.
3. The need for acceptance.
4. The need for privacy.
5. The need for a feeling of accomplishment.
6. The need for recognition and identity.
7. The need for belonging, for being wanted, for being needed.
8. The need for expression.

This week, pay attention to what you do or encourage during your time at the facility. What needs are you addressing? Which ones are left untouched? What could be done to provide your residents with a more full and satisfying day?

TODAY: Review needs.

Clinicians talk about the seven stages of Alzheimer's. Stage six, on paper, sounds almost fun—you don't care what others think; you do the first thing that pops into your head.

Somewhere during the middle stages of the disease, the dementia victim stops being able to dress herself. The task becomes enormously complicated, far too much for her to handle. In many nursing facilities, this stage signals a drastic change in wardrobe. Into the boxes go the clothes; out come the hospital johnnies. Staff don't have time to dress an uncooperative patient. Already having lost her memories, her skills and her connections to the present, the patient now loses her very wardrobe.

For Michael Warren, a CNA and an Alzheimer's consultant from Bellows Falls, stripping his patients of their personal clothing was not acceptable. An incredibly creative man, he devised a simple, cost effective method for maintaining his patients in their familiar outfits.

Each night Michael would take a few dresses home with him. He split each dress up the back, installed Velcro fasteners and, voila! An attractive, dignified johnny.

TODAY: Design creative accommodations.

Who are the writers in your building—not just letter writers, but the poets and storytellers? Every staff has someone who is gifted with a pen; surely there are a few residents who enjoy writing recollections and poetry.

This month get some of these amateur authors together and encourage them to publish a facility newsletter. If you already have a newsletter, then just convince these folks to contribute some of their writing.

At the Gill Home in Ludlow they produce an award-winning newsletter. Why is it award-winning? Because it is designed with the resident in mind. Some facilities focus on using the newsletter as a marketing tool with the general public or an information sheet for family members and responsible parties. The Gill newsletter is aimed at the people who live at the home. And because it is so well done, it ends up being a marketing tool and family news sheet anyway.

One of the highlights of each issue is the memory piece written by Evelyn Wilkins, a resident. Her reflections on days gone by are fascinating. Furthermore, the staff wisely publish with large print, again making it resident-friendly.

TODAY: Publish a resident-friendly newsletter.

Jan Haggerlin was an amazing staff person. Now living in Florida, Jan served for some time as activities director at Maple Lane Nursing Home.

A fairly new resident had been admitted to the facility, blind and in restraints. The hospital had apparently restrained her—a practice we have found quite common. It seems that hospitals often transfer such patients to nursing homes in restraints. When there are no documents which state the contrary, many facilities keep the restraints on, assuming that they are a long standing treatment.

Working with the rest of the staff, Jan was convinced that the belt restraint was unnecessary. Blind, this lady wasn't about to walk anywhere without some help.

With the restraint off, the patient got stronger and was able to walk with assistance. This terrific progress led Jan to ask the next logical question: "Why can't Mrs. Benson see?"

A trip to the eye doctor revealed the need for cataract surgery. The surgery was scheduled and successfully completed within a few weeks. As Mrs. Benson's bandages were removed, Jan quickly grabbed a colorful video cover and held it up. "Can you see this picture?" she asked.

"It looks like a bird," Mrs. Benson said.

Even a bird watcher couldn't have been as excited as Jan Haggerlin with Mrs. Benson's description of the Woody Woodpecker cartoon. She could see!

TODAY: Believe in the impossible.

Like it or not, our bodies do change dramatically as we age. Even at thirty and forty we don't look like we did in our teens and twenties. Gravity does have its way.

Yet I believe we all make a huge mistake if we imagine that, because the body isn't what it used to be, an individual loses his or her sexual appetite.

More than a few women and men in their eighties have confided to me about their escapades in the bedroom. Hooray for signs of life!

Nursing facility staff who are aware of this healthy aspect of their residents' lives can have some fun planning activities that tap into this natural energy and interest.

Such was the attitude that provoked a northern Vermont nursing facility to invite the famous Chippendale dancers to perform. And perform, in fact, the gorgeous, tan hunks did! On their next tour of New England, they fit an afternoon in at the facility, danced and posed for pictures with the residents.

Another home regularly books belly dancers for Father's Day, and even fathers who don't live at the institution drop by!

Tasteful, playful attention between men and women makes the world go 'round. Don't let your home be without it.

TODAY: Be aware of healthy signs of life.

No nursing facility I know of has a waiting list of people who want to work as nurses' aides. Let's face it—taking care of old people in the most intimate situations is not a glamorous job.

Where will the caregivers of the future come from?

Reading the wretched news, seeing the bloody television, listening to my son's stories of teenage life, I begin to feel our society is doomed.

The last time I heard such a discouraging word, I received this letter in the mail:

Dear Nursing Home:

I am sending you this money to buy anything you need for the people in your nursing home. I only want people to be happy. From Lauren, age 8.

P. S. It would make me happy if you used it on something for amusement for the people in the home.

Enclosed was a one dollar bill.

TODAY: Look for Laurens!

My friend Janet, a nurse, likes to talk about some of the silly things she was taught in nursing school. One day she was telling me about the time the class was studying DNA, and the instructor told them what certain chromosomes were responsible for, such as the color of eyes and hair and so forth. "At one point he said that there were several chromosomes with no use; they were just there," Janet recalled laughing.

Later in life, Janet said she realized that it wasn't that the chromosomes had no purpose; it was just that we humans haven't figured out their use yet.

When I heard the story of Pete and Elizabeth Davis of Liberty, S.C., I decided their chromosomes had something to do with it.

A devoted couple, they had always said they wanted to die at the same time. In January, 1993, both ninety-one, they died within seconds of each other on New Year's Eve, the day they would have celebrated their 69th wedding anniversary.

The newspaper account stated that "Mrs. Davis had health problems several years before her death, and the doctors suggested she move into a nursing home. Mr. Davis wouldn't let his wife go without him, and the two went to live in the nursing home in 1990, together."

What makes this story more sweet and fascinating is that Mr. Davis was in a coma when his wife died. The nurses think they heard Mrs. Davis stop breathing, and then Pete made his last gasp.

TODAY: Be in awe of the unknown.

Sometimes the sheer volume of the work can over-whelm you.

Think of bathing, dressing, feeding, walking and toileting a hundred or more patients a day. The laundry alone is staggering—hundreds of pounds a day. It is a noble calling to be committed to having the day be more than the basics. Getting through the day itself seems like plenty, without adding some special projects and programs.

Paul, a young, innovative administrator, did not have a nursing background. A business administration major, he had grown up around nursing homes, visiting them with his mom when she volunteered.

But the population of patients was different from the group he remembered meeting when he was a kid. Those folks were more alert, able to play checkers, talk.

Looking around this facility, the second one he had been asked to manage, Paul said he was struck by the lack of meaning. With no particular plan for any given day, staff and residents just went through the motions.

"We just passed people around. We didn't know what to do with them," he said.

This insight inspired Paul to work with his staff and develop a comprehensive program for dementia patients. Working with a nationally recognized trainer, he went about transforming the facility into a model operation. No more passing people around and keeping them busy for busy's sake.

TODAY: Stop passing people around.

Listening to families telling about the pivotal event that had brought their grandmothers to the nursing facility, broken hips seem to be at the top of the chart. So often a hip breaks and all other body functions begin to fail.

Because of the giant ramifications a broken hip can cause, staff are always trying to prevent falls. One of most common and dangerous places for falls is the bed with side rails. A confused resident needs to use the bathroom, crawls over the bed rails and falls onto the floor.

The bed rails, installed for safety, end up being the weapon.

At the Arbors, a nursing facility and residential care facility in Burlington, staff were particularly concerned about potential bedtime falls. All of the Arbors' residents have Alzheimer's or a related dementia, so nighttime wandering is a common occurrence.

One school of thought suggests that it is actually safer not to put the bed rails up. But the Arbors staff did not subscribe to that philosophy.

Clever brainstorming produced an unusual solution—futons. The futon, a Chinese cotton mattress, sits right on the floor. If the resident rolls out of bed, it is a gentle descent of about four inches. If someone wants to go walking, she or he must be able to stand up independently. Nighttime falls and wandering are almost eliminated by the futons.

TODAY: Produce unusual solutions.

Speaking in generalizations, in our civilization it is good to be young and bad to be old.

This narrow and nutty belief is the polar opposite of what older, more established cultures hold to be true. In the Asian world, to be old is to be revered. The oldest member of the family claims the position of authority and power in China, a custom more than 3,000 years old. In Japan, this same attitude prevails. Each year the Japanese declare one day to be Respect for the Aged Day, when all banks, schools and work places are closed. Citizens observe this holiday as a special and sacred day.

Among the Yanomamo tribe of South America, after an old relative dies, the remaining loved ones cremate the body. The bones are ground to a powder and mixed with a liquid. All who loved the deceased drink of this beverage, believing it honors and links their spirits.

TODAY: Declare today Respect for the Aged Day.

Frank had well earned the label "cantankerous." A widower in his nineties, Frank lived in a trailer on the edge of a farm and did things his way. He was unbelievably deaf and thus had mastered the one way conversation. There was no need to answer him: Frank could talk to himself, even on the phone.

In fact, Frank's phone calls were the very actions that had forced some civic leaders to make a decision. "Frank can't live alone anymore," the banker declared. "Frank needs to be with other people," the minister said. "Frank must have some nutritious meals," the senior citizens director added.

So the three local authorities drove up to Frank's trailer one day and asked him if he wanted to take a ride. Frank always wanted to a take a ride, especially to get to the store to buy some more White Owl cigars.

While the banker listened to a one way conversation from Frank, the other two hurriedly and secretly packed a large suitcase of clothes and stuck them in the trunk of the car. The drive ended at a retirement home, which just happened to have a room ready for Frank. The trio produced his suitcase, made some excuses, and disappeared.

Frank, ninety-four, was more than miserable—he was angry. He walked three miles to mail a letter to the town council. "Help! I've been kidnapped," it began.

Eventually I was handed the letter and went to meet Frank. Learning he had no guardian, that Frank was his own man, I took him back to his home where he showed me why he needed to live and die in his trailer. "Look in that closet," he motioned. Hanging neatly was a black suit, complete with shirt, tie and even socks tucked in the shoes.

"That's my burial suit. I'm going to die here, and I want them to dress me in that."

Frank lived two more years in his little trailer before he died, enjoying his cigars, baking homemade biscuits and washing windows on a step ladder.

TODAY: Be wary of the well-intentioned.

At age 102, Joe Hawkins, a honkytonk pianist from Augusta, GA, wrote this poem:

I've dreamed many dreams
　　that never came true,
I've seen them vanish at dawn.
But I've realized enough
　　of my dreams, thank God,
To make me want to dream on.

I've prayed many prayers
　　when no answer came,
Though I waited patient and long.
But enough answers have come
　　to enough of my prayers
To make me keep praying on.

I've trusted many
　　a friend that failed
And left me to weep alone.
But I've found enough
　　of my friends true blue
To make me keep trusting on.

I've sown many seeds
　　that fell by the way
For the birds to feed upon.
But I've held enough
　　golden sheaves in my hands,
To make me keep sowing on.

I've drained the cup
　　of disappointment and pain
And gone many days without song.

But I've sipped enough nectar
   from the roses of life
To make me want to live on.

TODAY: Read Joe's poem to your patients.

Gary had worked as a nurses' aide long enough to know what a bad day looked like. Starting out overtired, finding his wing short-staffed, Gary's day took a downhill slide.

Exhausted and unable to look on the bright side and see anything, Gary went into a tailspin. No matter what might happen, he saw the worst. Everything stank.

Working the three to eleven shift, he was anxious to just get those people in bed and asleep. No more requests, complaints, or craziness.

Duke was never an easy patient, and Gary was in no mood for his usual guff. But tonight, Duke was pleasant and easy going, almost as if he sensed Gary needed a break. As Gary pulled up the covers on Duke and turned on his fan, Duke said hoarsely, "Good night. I love you."

On his drive home that night, Gary said he realized "A good night makes up for a bad day."

TODAY: Look for turning points.

A man who had been for seven years the full-time chaplain of a nursing home published an article in the AARP magazine about the merit of using CPR in nursing homes. He wrote:

> My teachers have been little old ladies in their eighties, their loving families and scores of caring nurses. Here is where I am today.

> I believe the evidence is overwhelming showing the futility of CPR on the frail, ill, elderly nursing home resident....CPR in this setting only contributes to the prolonging of the dying process. The one successful use of CPR I have seen in this situation revived a woman suffering from emphysema. After her resuscitation she lived the final weeks of her life struggling for every breath.

> Though convinced of its futility, I will defend anyone's right to receive CPR. I have taken CPR training and stand ready to administer it to any resident who wants it. The key idea here is what is the wish of the resident. Over and over I have asked residents, "If your heart were to stop would you want the nurses to attempt to restart it?" Most say "No. Let me go in peace."

TODAY: Know your patients' wishes.

Mrs. Blow was a born saleswoman. It mattered little that she was well over eighty and living in a nursing facility. She was put on the planet to sell, and sell she did.

The smart staff knew sales was what Mrs. Blow was all about. The activities program always received donations of castoffs and always needed money. So, just about every afternoon, five days a week, you would find Mrs. Blow setting up her card table in the hallway, selling the donated goods that weren't wanted and raising money for wanted goods. She also sold crafts made, at times, by other residents.

Nobody tried to walk by Mrs. Blow without buying. Why, she would already have something picked out for you! And during the Chamber of Commerce raffles, she was happy to sell you five tickets at a time. After all, last year she sold the winning ticket to a woman who just happened to drop by. "Might be your turn this year," she would say with her saleswoman-style smile. So, we all bought.

TODAY: Use your sales people!

Some nursing facilities seem to have a plantation mentality. There is the big boss man (the administrator), and everyone else is considered some kind of slave. Some of the slaves are in charge of other slaves, but they are still slaves.

Okay, so I'm a little harsh and dramatic here. Maybe not slavery, but certainly not total equality either. I am both angered and saddened when I visit homes where this kind of staff caste-system exists.

Like the home where management got free coffee, and CNAs had to buy their coffee out of a machine. Or the building where there was no heat in the staff lounge. And then there was the home that, when holding a meeting for visiting managers, served cheese, fruit, shrimp and hot rolls. (For a gathering of nurses' aides, the menu was red powdered drink and crackers.) At yet another facility, the only air-conditioned room is the administrator's office, though the kitchen gets close to a hundred degrees in the summer.

Not only does such a primitive way of treating people degrade staff, it affects the lives of the patients too. After all, if you're a staff person who has been reminded all day that you are low person on the totem pole, wouldn't you sometimes want to feel bigger than someone else? Maybe lord some power over a helpless patient?

Power and responsibility is best exercised when it is shared. Resist the temptation to look down on anyone. Everyone has worth and value.

TODAY: Treat others as equals.

We're all dying, some of us seem readier than others.

For some of your residents, their last breath will be a sigh of relief. They have suffered mightily.

Some of the staff act half dead now, dragging around in an angry fog, quick to tell you what's wrong with this stinking place, unable to sing praises or bring joy.

Today, in fact, is not only the first day of the rest of your life, it could be your last. For all that we feel we know about life, we can't predict our death.

Given the fleeting, precious nature of life, why not set today aside for simply appreciating? For just observing the beauty around you and little else? Treat your eyes, spirit and heart to a good time.

Linden Lodge (Brattleboro) dedicated its Summer 1987 issue of the Linden Ledger to that "Enviable capacity we sometimes see in others—to enjoy and appreciate life while we live it, each and every minute." The front page article continued:

> Bask in the summer sunshine; relish the rich diversity in the faces you encounter today; delight in the colors of your surroundings; lend your ear to the vibrant sounds of life; brush a flower with your fingertips; breathe deeply of its fragrance; flex a muscle; hum a tune; laugh; weep, sigh; smile! In this very moment lies all the tangible peace and beauty of life itself. Grasp it to yourself, then fling it in joy to the first person you meet! We call this LIFE-RELISHMENT and we wish you an abundant and inexhaustible supply of the same!

TODAY: Practice life-relishment.

What's it like to be a stranger at your facility? When a visitor walks through the door, what happens?

If we think of ourselves as being caring members of a close community, bound together by a commitment to quality and compassion, our instinct will be to greet guests warmly.

"Hello, I'm Bethany, a nursing assistant. Can I help you?"

The relief on the visitor's face will be immediate. Everyone wants to feel welcome and at ease. All too often, for many reasons, new people walk through the front door of the facility and wander around self-consciously, trying to find the office, the kitchen, their friend. Too shy or too proud to ask directions, they wander around hoping they'll figure something out.

Staff and residents stare at the stranger, sometimes with suspicion. The already tense visitor gets even more uptight.

From a security standpoint, it is just plain smart to talk with unfamiliar faces and find out what they are doing in your building. The world is full of all kinds of people, and some types absolutely do not belong in a nursing facility. Being friendly is wise and wonderful. Don't assume anything about visitors. Say "hello" and go from there.

TODAY: Greet strangers.

Ask any caregiver about the first time they bathed a patient and you'll get a smile or a giggle. No doubt about it, such intimate contact with another adult is something you gradually adjust to. Of course it feels odd; bathing is a private matter.

Jean was a pretty shy nurses' aide. Her family was modest, and she had not grown up with nudity. Even her sister had never undressed in front of her. Jean took her work very seriously and often anguished about giving a new patient a bath. She would offer to do anything else for a coworker, if she would just bathe the new woman in room 302.

One morning Jean was scheduled to give a sponge bath to Mrs. Dylan, a bedridden woman who had been transferred from the hospital only the day before. Jean had talked a little with her yesterday, but today she had to take the plunge and get her feet (and hands!) wet.

Taking things step by step, Jean worked hard to be calm, making small talk as she washed Mrs. Dylan. Can you imagine Jean's disbelief when she discovered, while taking care of her peri area, that Mrs. Dylan was once Mr. Dylan? It seems this woman, now in her seventies, had a sex-change operation years ago, switching from he to she. Jean knew she had seen everything now!

TODAY: Expect the unexpected.

Given their average life spans, there aren't many men in long term care facilities. Basically, it's a woman's world—female patients and staff.

Joe Bennett was one of only a handful of men at the home. A dairy farmer in his eighties, Joe had survived a terrible accident that had left him paralyzed and in a wheelchair.

When Joe was in his late seventies, he had climbed a ladder to knock ice dams off his roof. For more than fifty years Joe had cracked these thick blocks of ice off the eaves to prevent melting water from ruining his ceilings and walls. No one knows why that particular March morning Joe lost his footing.

He can't remember much except that the mailman found him more than twenty-four hours later, after he had lain in the snow and the cold overnight. A bachelor, he had no family who checked on him.

More than ten surgeries later, Joe had the use of his upper body. Always a robust, physically active man, he considered the wheelchair his prison. "This is hell!" he would say to anyone who would listen. "I wish that damn mailman hadn't found me."

No matter what the activities department suggested, Joe would have no part of any programs or projects. "Stupid social stuff," he would mutter, staring out the window. When he first came to the home, he talked about returning to his farm. He didn't do that anymore.

One day a young drawing teacher came to the facility, and Joe said his usual "nope" to the idea. "Drawing is for sissies, for girls!" he said firmly.

But the gentle teacher persisted, asking Joe to tell him about life on the farm. After a while, Joe began to talk with real enthusiasm about all the buildings he had erected. "Built four barns on my own property and helped build ten others," he would boast.

"I've never built a barn," the drawing teacher confessed. "Can you draw for me how it's done?"

So began Joe Bennett's artistic career. He spent a good year on drawing buildings until, one day, he added the landscape. Now he dabbles in still lifes, portraits, collages. He draws up to four hours a day and enjoys every minute.

TODAY: Discover artists!

A most unusual group of nursing homes operates in South Dakota, and it is run by a most unusual man.

On his resumé you will find him listed as Dr. Mark A. Jerstad, chief executive officer of The Evangelical Lutheran Good Samaritan Society. He holds a doctoral degree and began his professional life as a campus pastor and professor of religion.

So how did he end up directing a large nursing home business? In 1984 Dr. Jerstad took some time off from his college duties to enroll in an administrator-in-training program with the Good Samaritan Society nursing homes. His plan was very simple. He hoped to develop a possible program in gerontology and long term care at the college.

But, as he wrote in Provider magazine (June, 1995), "It proved to be a life-changing experience."

Dr. Jerstad shares one of his journal entries from this time:

> Wow! I have been here for two weeks and I am overwhelmed—overwhelmed with the warmth of love, struggles, great humor and deep commitment of the staff.

Explaining his move from higher education to health care, Dr. Jerstad writes:

Though I had intended only a short break from the Augustana campus, I found myself captured by a labor of love that would challenge me for a lifetime. I joined the Good Samaritan Society full time in 1985. I have spent countless hours in nursing facilities across the country. In every facility, I have witnessed the dramatic way in which nurse assistants and other front line staff can change the quality of life for those we serve.

TODAY: Appreciate management.

Hot August days can be the perfect time to organize a drive in the country.

It's amazing how many people own neat old cars. Sometimes they are genuine antiques (twenty-five years or older) and sometimes they are just well maintained convertibles, trucks or even dune buggies.

Getting out of the facility and going for a nice drive, with no destination or errands, can be a grand boost to the morale. Remember those nights you took one of your colicky babies for a ride, hoping he or she would finally fall asleep? Car rides are good for the soul; we all like to feel that hum and see the world go by.

At Brookside Nursing Home, someone's son drove up one day in a souped-up hot rod. For about two hours he shuttled passengers around the village for a little sightseeing and stimulation. Riders talked about that spin for at least a week.

Why not talk with other staffers and even visiting family members. Find out who is willing to be part of a little caravan this week.

TODAY: Organize a drive.

Coming home at the end of the work day, we all face even more responsibilities. Meals, laundry and cleaning all call our name. Often, after a tough day, the last thing we want to do is more.

Roger Beaudoin, a nurses' aide at McKerley healthcare Center in Bedford, New Hampshire, is no different from the rest of us. He too is tired, aching and pretty foggy when he gets home.

Yet Roger takes time to write poetry—about work.

One of his best is a forty-eight line piece called "Life of a Nurses' Aide." Here are the last sixteen lines:

> I pull some muscles in my back
> From lifting that I do
> And I'm a friend to those who lack
> And I'm a mother too
> I'm always giving love and care
> In work that I perform
> And to each one who's lying there
> A gentle touch so warm
> A healthcare center couldn't run
> Or service those in need
> If not for every special one
> Who works so hard indeed
> No words could ever truly state
> The contributions made
> And valued service very great
> By every nurses' aide.

TODAY: Write a poem about work.

August 27

Once a month, usually the first Wednesday of the month, it's Donut Day at Berlin Health and Rehabilitation Center.

Only people who haven't stopped by BHRC on Donut Day need to ask what it is. Once you've been to a Donut Day, you'll never forget it and you'll probably never miss another either.

Pam Prue, assistant activities director, heads up the donut-making crew of some ten to twelve residents and two or three volunteers. Pam comes from a family of nine kids and her mom taught her to cook for crowds.

Imagine you're sitting with the assistant donut makers around the huge square table. Everyone has a job: stirring the baking powder into the milk, beating the eggs, mixing the milk and eggs, adding the flour. Lots of mixing bowls in laps; flour flying; baking stories bubbling over. The best part is, of course, the eating. Donuts are delivered to all 158 residents, warm and delicious. Staff can buy them by the dozen.

Pam's Mother's Donuts

3 c. sugar	2 c. milk
4 T. lard, melted	2 heaping t. baking powder for each c. milk
1 t. mace	
1 1/2 t. nutmeg	7 c. flour (6 and 1) 6 c. in batter, 1 c. on table for kneading (more flour may be needed for batter)
1 t. salt	
1/4 t. cinnamon	
1 t. vanilla	
4 eggs	

Mix, sugar and lard well. Combine and mix mace (the secret ingredient!), nutmeg, salt, cinnamon and vanilla and add to first mixture. Mix eggs in small bowl first, then add to batter. Put 2 heaping teaspoons baking powder in 1 cup milk and stir. Add quickly to batter. Add 2 more heaping teaspoons baking powder in 2nd cup milk and stir and add to batter. Add flour and fold in. Mix with hands. Do not roll out! Knead and pat to 1/4 inch thickness. Cut with donut cutter. Deep fry in 4 to 5 lbs. hot lard or Crisco for a few minutes on each side (golden) turning with chopsticks only once. Drain on paper towels. Powder or cinnamon sugar in plastic bags, optional.

TODAY: Swap recipes.

Families vacationing in the area sometimes drop by the facility for a surprise summer visit. Full of guilt, they think they have to bring gifts and suggest a big outing.

If you know your patients well, you know who would genuinely enjoy an outing and who hates leaving her room. Helping families do what's best for their loved one is an art.

Too frequently staff will guilt-trip the weak patient, thinking they are being helpful: "Now, Margaret, your children came a long way. You don't want them to feel bad, do you?" Poor Margaret, then, cannot think of how she feels, but must think of her healthy grown children's hurt feelings.

I once watched Karen, the activities director, walk through the small McGirr's Nursing Home in Bellows Falls on a hot summer afternoon. "Who wants to go for a ride in the van for some ice cream?" she sang out up and down the halls. Her enthusiasm was met with gracious "no thank you's." Everyone had their reasons, but they all could be translated into one sentence: "I don't want to."

My favorite response came from a gentle, wispy lady who looked up from her nap. "I don't want any, dear. But why don't you go and treat yourself?" Karen respected what the patients told her, never wheedling or guilt-tripping anyone.

TODAY: Respect resident's wishes.

Reading the obituaries, I am always moved by what people consider important and worth mentioning in the last roundup on their lives.

The expected includes family, from parents to wife to children and grandchildren. Work and hobbies are usually included, as are memberships. Once in a while something special will be noted. "He was named Boss of the Year by the Rotary in 1957."

Being named Boss of the Year is a big deal. Think how many bosses there are and how many are horrible! If you have a supervisor who is fair, appreciative and encouraging, why not nominate him or her for an award?

Most communities, through the Rotary Club, Chamber of Commerce, or some other professional organization, have such a competition. Call the public library; they can tell you. And if your city doesn't have any awards program, why not start one? And make sure your boss is the first winner!

At the very least, you can write a letter to the editor of the local paper and get the rest of the staff to sign it. Tell your town what a great boss you have.

TODAY: Pat your boss on the back.

The Scouts have a motto: Be Prepared.

Most schools have mottoes. The Marines proclaim Semper Fidelis ("Always Faithful"). Burger King declares "Have it your way!" and KFC says "We do chicken right!"

What is the motto of your nursing facility?

If your home is like most, you haven't selected your motto yet. It's time for a contest, asking staff and residents to suggest sayings or statements that your home lives up to.

Hospice programs generally have a statement of purpose, which is like a motto. One common one is "We add life to days when days can no longer be added to life."

One home has a theme song, sung at the end of virtually every event: "One day at a time, sweet Jesus, that's all I'm asking of you," the lyrics go. No matter what the occasion, the song fits.

TODAY: Write your motto.

Old Ned couldn't live alone anymore. He had left the eggs boiling on the stove for so long that they blew up and the aluminum pan melted into the burner. He got confused a lot and even went out one night after midnight, walking down the center of the road, naked, to the school board meeting.

His younger brother Bob finally got Ned into a nursing home just a few blocks from their family church. Ned wasn't happy, but he wasn't able to manage alone anymore either.

The nurses and aides doted on Ned. He had been the town constable, and everyone knew the old coot. Almost a pet patient, Ned seemed to always have staff swarming around him. One day, as he tipped to one side and then the other in his wheelchair, a nurse rushed over and said "Ned! Let me readjust your pillows. We don't want you leaning over and getting stiff."

His faithful brother Bob visited that day, as he had each day for two months, checking on how Ned was being treated. Bob asked Ned the usual "How's everything?" and Ned, instead of his customary "fine," said "Well, I do have a problem."

Bob, troubled, asked, "What?"

"Well," old Ned began, "they're always all around me; they won't leave me alone. Why this afternoon they were so darn worried I was tipping over in my chair they wouldn't even let me pass gas!"

TODAY: Don't over-dote.

September

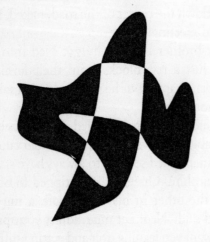

Every day, the newspaper, radio and television report on the rising costs of health care. The phrases "health care" and "cost effective" seem to be partners for life.

Hospitals are particularly scrutinized for costly procedures and equipment purchases. High-tech surgery and transplants cause healthcare bills and insurance premiums to be constantly on the rise.

Nursing homes don't provide sophisticated medical procedures, yet a concern about cost effectiveness is still very present. Staff efficiency and productivity are closely watched, always with the hope that time can be trimmed and more services delivered for the same price.

Often, in the name of efficiency, a patient's wishes or needs can be overlooked. Feeding people in their rooms means less time is spent walking to the dining hall, but does the patient have enough changes in scenery?

Sometimes, in the rush to get everybody up and out, an aide will sacrifice the little somethings that make life so much nicer. Small talk, jokes and stories can make the day so much brighter. Ask any patient— they would prefer special attention over efficiency any day.

TODAY: Take time to be you.

Losing a loved one is a life changing experience. As time passes the loss may lose its sting, but it never becomes easy or okay. Our mother, father, or daughter is dead. That is what remains.

When a loved one becomes a victim of dementia, the loss is also painful and powerful. Some say it is even worse than death, as the person is still physically present.

To deal with losing her grandmother to Alzheimer's and a nursing home, ten-year-old Hannah Peck (of Putney) wrote a poem entitled "Distance and Bama."

In part, Hannah wrote:

A wall of mist
Is keeping us separate
That's all
It's as if she wished to know me
But can't.
Sometimes a smile
Will spread cross her wrinkling face
Smiling at me
Like the mist had broken
Just for a minute
Not long enough.

Even in her weakened state, Hannah's grandmother is providing for Hannah. She is inspiring her to write poetry, good poetry, at ten years of age.

TODAY: See how families rise above pain.

The American way of life means one's identity is closely linked to work; upon introduction, people usually ask each other, "What's your name?" and "What do you do?"

For the unemployed and retired, this work-worshipping society can be tough to live in. For those in nursing facilities, it can mean having almost no identity at all. Duncan Robb, a social worker at Central Vermont Hospital in Berlin, gave this statement by an anonymous author:

> The real curse of being old is the ejection from a citizenship traditionally based on work… It is a demeaning idleness, nonuse, not being called on any longer to contribute and hence being put down as a spent person of no public account.

Early in September we celebrate the Labor Day holiday, honoring working men and women. This year why not hold some special ceremony recognizing the work histories of your residents? Add up the years they, as a group, have worked, and put that many hundreds of candles on cakes. Or give them each a cake with his or her own number of years. Then group the former homemakers, teachers and nurses together. Bring in young people who are just entering those professions to talk with them about the way the work used to be.

Our nation, states and communities all were kept going with the hard work and tax dollars of the people who now live in your facility. Keep this thought in mind and give them the respect they deserve.

 TODAY: Respect the work lives of residents.

Exaggeration and hyperbole are sure signs of human nature. Animals don't embellish their stories to each other; only the talking human being can do that.

The one that got away becomes bigger every time a fisherman tells the story. And so does the jackpot you only missed by one number.

Such embroidery of the truth, as my father used to call it, does serve a purpose. For whatever reason, people need to make their lives sound a little better, a little fancier, a little more amazing than they actually were. When we give our own spin to our lives, we somehow can live with pain and disappointment better.

Listening to your patients tell and retell their life stories, you can hear the extra touches.

James Thurber captures this habit in his charming fable *The Moth and the Star*. The story goes that a young moth set his heart on a certain star. His brothers and sisters all set their sights on reachable, nearby bridge-lamps. His parents kept telling him he wouldn't get anywhere chasing stars, but he didn't listen. Thurber writes:

The moth left his father's house, but he would not fly around street lamps and he would not fly around house lamps. He went right on trying to reach the star, which was four and one-third light years, or twenty-five trillion miles, away. The moth thought it was just caught in the top branches of an elm. He never did reach the star, but went right on trying, night after night, and when he was a very, very old moth he began to think that he really had reached the star and he went around saying so. This gave him a deep and lasting pleasure, and he lived to a great old age. His parents and his brothers and his sisters had all been burned to death when they were quite young.

MORAL: Who flies afar from the sphere of our sorrow is here today and here tomorrow.

TODAY: Listen to star stories.

September 5

At the weekly worship service in the facility sun room, a mere handful of women over ninety sat in a semicircle. At the closing prayer, the chaplain asked for the names of those who needed special prayers.

Mable asked for prayers for her ears and lower back; Bertha, for better vision, her friend facing surgery and all the hungry people in the world; Carol, for her friends with Alzheimer's and the wars being fought on our planet; Laura, for her brother's swift recovery from surgery.

When it came to ninety-eight-year-old Madge, she said, "I can't think of anything, thank you." The chaplain jumped in: "Isn't that wonderful? Everything is okay, then?"

"Oh, no! Everything isn't okay," Madge responded, startled. "I've just accepted what is."

Following Madge, Florence asked for prayers of thanksgiving for her many blessings.

What an exquisite demonstration of the range of prayer! Our supplications can rightly be for the healing of self, for loved ones, for mankind in total. And we can pray for the strength to accept what can't be changed and for the grace to appreciate our good fortune.

Sounds like the ladies wrote their own Serenity Prayer, huh?

TODAY: Accept what is.

Thinking big can be a smart way to live. Setting high goals and standards can push us into great achievements. Look at the Olympic athletes and what they have accomplished!

Thinking big when it comes to delivering services to needy people can also be smart. Buying in bulk or quantity always saves money. While one home health nurse can only visit seven or eight patients a day in their private homes, a nursing home nurse can visit fifty or more patients.

Still, for all the benefits of the cost effective institutional setting, there are some disadvantages to consider too.

Samuel Gridley Howe of Boston is credited with spearheading the drive to establish the first state operated residential facility in the US in 1866.

In looking back on the creation of these state residences for the masses, we can see that Howe developed some general principles which should underlie all such establishments. He was especially concerned with the tendency to isolate populations with their own kind. His belief was that the institutionalized should not be segregated.

He wrote:

> As much as may be, surround insane and excitable persons with sane people and ordinary influences; vicious children with virtuous people and virtuous influences; blind children with those who see; mute children with those who speak; and the like.

Howe also recommended that we keep institutions as small as we can.

As you group your patients together for meals and activities, consider Howe's words. Do you agree? Disagree? Organize a discussion, or even a debate, at one of your staff meetings. What do your colleagues think is the best arrangement?

TODAY: Special units: to be or not to be?

The great truths are always very basic. Know thyself. Do unto others as you would have others do unto you. Look both ways.

Being in a good mood makes life easier. That's a great, basic truth. No matter how good your reasons are for being mad, grouchy, sad, or numb, they can't compete with the superiority of being in a good mood.

Of course, experiencing a tragedy is not something we can pop out of in an hour or a day or even a week. We all need time to heal and accept our terrible loss.

Bad moods brought on by stupid things are so unnecessary, and yet they are a common cause of suffering.

Saskia Davis recommends we choose a different kind of suffering—suffering from inner peace. What are the symptoms of this malady?

A tendency to think and act spontaneously rather than on fears based on past experiences.

An unmistakable ability to enjoy each moment.

A loss of interest in judging other people.

A loss of interest in judging self.

A loss of interest in interpreting the actions of others.

A loss of interest in conflict.

A loss of the ability to worry. (This is a serious symptom.)

Frequent, overwhelming episodes of appreciation.

Contented feelings of connectedness with others and nature.

Frequent attacks of smiling through the eyes from the heart.

An increasing tendency to let things happen rather than make them happen.

An increased susceptibility to the love extended by others as well as the uncontrollable urge to extend it.

TODAY: Suffer inner peace.

Is there anything harder than watching a crummy family let down one of your patients?

Jeanine's patient Angela was dying. The family, though they lived less than five miles away, never came to visit. Because of Angela's condition, the social worker called and encouraged them to drop by.

About a week later, Angela's older son and his wife arrived. By this time Angela was in and out of consciousness. After a short visit, her daughter-in-law looked around the room and, taking a beautiful crystal lamp, said, "Well, mom won't be needing this anymore."

In the days that followed, other family members came and cleaned out the room of all personal things. Jeanine watched in horror, as it became clear the visits were really opportunities to pick up family heirlooms, not to visit family.

On the day Angela died, Jeanine was alone with her. No family came. The room had been picked clean.

"They sure gave me a good lesson about stuff," Jeanine said later. "Things just aren't important—people are. They never saw that."

TODAY: Find lessons every day.

Bob Sterling, administrator of Green Mountain Nursing Home in Colchester, believes in the trickle-down theory. And he puts his money where his mouth is.

When his facility had a state inspection that resulted in only two minor deficiencies, he decided the entire staff, from chief cook to bottle washer, and everyone in between, should be rewarded.

Working quietly with his bookkeeper, Bob bought $50 savings bonds for each and every employee. That next payday, when staff people came to the office to pick up their checks, the bookkeeper would say, "Oh, Mr. Sterling wants to see you."

Sitting at his desk, Bob thanked each employee for his or her contribution to the facility's exceptional survey. He then presented them with a savings bond.

TODAY: Show this page to your boss!

Don't those crybaby employees who can't take any pain or discomfort drive you crazy?

Why, she cut herself and can't use her hand at all. He pulled a muscle playing softball and he's barely able to walk.

Being careful and letting our bodies heal is one thing. Being theatrical and milking our accidents well beyond their shelf life is another.

When it comes to overcoming an injury, don't whine to Angel Wallenda. A member of the Flying Wallenda acrobatic team, this young mother was diagnosed with cancer in 1990. Her treatment included the amputation of a leg.

For someone who makes her living walking the high wire, the amputation could have easily meant the end of her career.

But one year after her diagnosis, fitted with a prosthetic leg, Angel walked the wire in front of the carving of Confederate leaders at Stone Mountain, GA. Her husband and five-year-old son watched. Don't complain to Angel about hardship.

TODAY: Overcome.

Who says old people confined in wheelchairs can't make a difference? Nobody at Verdelle Village in St. Albans!

When the administrator, Paul Richards, got involved with the American Heart Association, he knew he also wanted to involve the staff and residents of the facility. Paul knew a fund-raiser would be the most helpful project for the Association, but who had any money to donate?

Started in 1990, the annual Verdelle Wheelathon for the American Heart Association is an undeniable success. Residents and staff collect pledges from near and far, asking folks to donate a set amount of money for every time a wheelchair-bound resident travels once around the outside of the facility.

A regular race track is set up, with staff taking turns pushing residents. Along the way there are refreshment stands, first aid, even a hose for cooling off. A local radio station is at the finish line broadcasting live music and the play-by-play of the event. Donated foods from area merchants and dairies are also on hand.

Beyond the excitement and fun the Wheelathon generates, the funds raised are nothing to sneeze at. In 1993, Verdelle turned a check over to the Heart Association for $13,000.

A well-planned and well-worth-it event. What cause could your facility get behind?

TODAY: Adopt a cause.

Plenty of clichés fit this story:
What goes around, comes around.
The pendulum always swings back.
There's nothing new under the sun.

Yet despite the fact that the concept of primary care is well established in healthcare circles, it is fairly new to the nursing facility setting.

Primary care means staff are permanently assigned to the same patients. Because the facility does not switch daily the list of residents that an aide takes care of, permanent bonds are established. Hospitals have used this staffing model for a long time, while nursing facilities are only now seeing the value for both residents and staff.

Imagine being a frail, modest resident. How would you like having a different employee bathing you every day? How would you like, each time you went for a bath, having to explain to unfamiliar staff, "Please don't hold me that way because I have a bad shoulder"?

Primary care encourages relationships between caregiver and care receiver. The employee gets to know each one she is taking care of; she notices even the slightest changes in conditions. Regardless of the residents' health or well-being, they are never handed over to another staffer. Even when the final days come and death is near, the primary care team is present.

TODAY: Ask your supervisor about trying the primary care model.

No one's life is simple, one dimensional or without pain and suffering.

Working for years on the same job, one can develop a hardened shell, an attitude that says, "I've seen it all; I can do this work with my eyes closed." Patients become objects, just props in the facility.

Not only is this stagnant thinking sad, it is also dangerous. Accidents happen when we go to work on automatic pilot, thinking that no thinking is necessary.

To guard against this hardening of attitudes, caregivers need to remind themselves that behind every wrinkled, aging exterior lies a beating heart and a history. Each resident has had his or her share of secrets and shame; some have mysteries they are taking with them to the grave.

When Robert and Joyce went to their late mother's home in suburban Baltimore in February of 1989, their mission was to find her will and settle the estate. Neither of them expected what they found in the steamer trunk in the basement—the skeleton body of an infant girl clothed in a T-shirt that said "World's Fair 1939."

According to the medical examiner, the baby had lived for about one month and had died of an unknown cause about fifty years ago.

Martha C. Shields, aged sixty-seven years, died without telling that story. Who knows what grief and guilt she might have held inside for so many years. Who knows if her caregivers were able to provide her with any understanding, relief or counsel?

TODAY: Be ready for your patient's secrets.

Fancy textbooks refer to kids and patients getting together as "intergenerational activities." The kids in Mrs. Melancon's third grade and the residents of Cedar Hill Nursing Home in Windsor call it FUN!

From September to May of 1993, these two groups of people got together once a month, for parties, games, singing, crafts and just plain visiting. In a thank-you letter written by the class to the residents, beautiful memories were recalled. They wrote in part:

> We arrived that first day, and we were so shy. As the time passed, we talked and learned a lot about each other. It was hard for us to talk loud enough to be heard, but somehow you understood. And we did not always have to talk. Sometimes it was special just being beside you and seeing your smile. We were so excited when we left we could not wait until our next visit.
>
> April hopped onto our calendar and we colored Easter eggs with you. What beautiful eggs they were. It was so much fun. Your generosity did not stop there. Before we arrived you had made lovely Easter baskets for each one of us and filled them with candy and gum. You were so proud of the bunnies you had cut out and glued to the front of each basket. We were very grateful. Now we are such good friends that it is easy for us to put our arms around you for special pictures when we say goodbye.
>
> How do we express the feelings that have grown inside this past year? How do we express

the sense of loss we will feel when we have to say goodbye? You will remain in our hearts forever.

TODAY: Plan an intergenerational fun event!

Romance. Can anything beat it?

No matter what our age, circumstances or education, we all love to hear about love. Some of us may act like it is silly, goofy and hardly worth talking about. But we still want to hear about people falling in love.

In my lifetime I have heard of three romances that actually resulted in marriage at nursing homes. Each couple was precious and each nursing facility did its darnedest to make the weddings beautiful ceremonies.

When Bev and Hank got married, she was confined to a wheelchair. Hank had been visiting his wife at the nursing home for several years before she died. So accustomed to visiting the facility was he, that Hank continued to visit and drew closer and closer to his late wife's roommate. The rest is history written by Cupid. And as in the movie *An Officer and a Gentleman,* Hank took his new bride home with him.

Freda and Henry met, married and remained in the nursing facility. The director of nursing made her wedding gown; the kitchen prepared a beautiful reception. The staff redecorated a room for the couple and even moved in a double bed. For that honeymoon weekend, room service was delivered and visitors were kept at a distance.

When my friend, Tina Whalley, and I were rooming together at Duke for summer school, she learned her grandmother had fallen in love in a Virginia nursing home. "I'm getting married next week," her grandmother had written. Tina, who was licensed to perform weddings, would be back in less than two weeks.

Could her grandmother wait for Tina to marry her?
No! She had waited long enough to find her dream
man!

TODAY: Look for romance.

If you've ever lived away from home, you know how important mail and telephone calls become. I remember how much I treasured my letters from my father when I was at Girl Scout camp in the summer. Boy, they were so funny!

Such connections with the outside world, and especially with people we love, are just as important to people living in nursing homes. Just look at the birthday cards displayed on the window sill or on the bedside table. How many months old are they? Or the postcard from Florida tacked on the wall. How long ago did her granddaughter take that trip?

Knowing the special value of mail, it seems incredible that some nursing facilities can be so very lazy about delivery. Precious, personal letters can often sit for days on the social worker's desk as she tries to make time to bring them to room 101.

If you know of similar sloppy delays in getting the mail to your patients, do something about it. Organize a volunteer group of mail-delivery people, perhaps patients who are interested and able. The US Postal Service promises they will get it to the facility, regardless of rain, sleet, snow or hail. Don't let a little disorganization stop a letter at your home.

TODAY: Deliver de letter, de sooner, de better!

Little Arlene was so humble I almost overlooked her greatness. A soft-faced, white-haired lady, Arlene's eyes were failing rapidly. It seemed every week I saw her she was more unsure of herself.

A woman who had worked her whole life as a nurses' aide in the state mental hospital, Arlene was a gentle soul. It was hard to imagine her in an institution for the insane, she seemed so fragile and delicate.

A morning worship service had triggered some long forgotten pain in Arlene's past, and I was asked to go to her room. There I found Arlene in her chair, gazing out the window, weeping.

As her story unraveled, I learned how, over twenty years ago, her husband of some forty years had run off on Christmas Eve with her daughter's best friend. I learned how Arlene had been asked by a stranger to raise a four-year-old girl, which she did until the girl married and began her own family. Arlene's strength and compassion overwhelmed me. Like the ant who can lift 35 times his weight, Arlene had managed unbelievable circumstances with such grace and no bitterness!

We prayed together, and I thanked God for bringing us together. I also asked that Arlene see her own goodness and how much God loved her.

TODAY: Meet the giants in your world.

My friend Mikell, who has lived much of her life in and out of mental institutions and care homes, taught me about another sign of discrimination.

A beautiful woman, Mikell is always meticulously groomed—makeup, jewelry, her hair often in a colorful scarf.

At the drop-in center she occasionally visits, the bathrooms are not marked "men" and "women" as is usually the case. Instead they say "staff only" and "clients."

This distinction hurt Mikell; she made a point of mentioning it to the staff; she even wrote a little article about it for the program newsletter. To her, separating people in this fashion smacked of segregation, of the anti-black laws of the pre-civil rights South.

In our nursing facilities, similar labeling and division occurs. Much of it can be chalked up to "We've always done it that way." Little thought is invested in the reasons anymore. Probably no one thinks about the possibility that feelings are hurt.

Sure, if we want to we can crank out plenty of reasons (hygiene, privacy, efficiency) for staff-versus-resident bathrooms. But, as we justify our segregation, let's also spend a moment thinking about what such an us-versus-them policy does to keep people in their place.

TODAY: Evaluate your staff-only policies and space.

I love my friend Ruth. She is eighty-nine, was married to Russell for sixty-five years and worked in the schools all her working life. Her involvement with the Methodist Church runs deep and wide. A career choir member, she has supported the church in many capacities.

When we first met, I fell in love with her as she sang (mostly giggled) from the church choir one Sunday morning. Seems she had picked up the wrong sheet music, so she was "faking" the hymn without much success. Her cheery smile was that of an eight-year-old laughing at herself.

Ruth likes to talk about how she sold her bike only a few years ago and about the vigorous life she led as a schoolteacher, mother and wife. Now, with plenty of maladies, she limits herself to crocheting huge numbers of afghans, all of which go to charity. When we drop over for a visit, and she talks about her hiatal hernia, or her very sore back, she always adds, "It's this darned old lady business!"

I love the expression, not just because it is of Ruth, but because it is such a clear example of how important it is to remember we aren't our diseases or disabilities. In her spirit, Ruth is still eight years old, singing and riding her bike. The fact that her body isn't cooperating is a nuisance, but Ruth doesn't see it as changing the person she knows herself to be. Her problems aren't really about being Ruth; they are just that "darned old lady business."

TODAY: Keep that darned old lady business in its place.

Insurance salesmen who want to be country western singers, nurses who long to be journalists, carpenters who want to be photographers—so many of us harbor fantasy identities, thinking we're not good enough in what we're doing, thinking we aren't making a difference.

Buddy is the finest chef I have ever met. He serves more than 500 meals a day to people with all kinds of special diets and restrictions. He doesn't just rotate the same menu every month; he creates in his kitchen. I have attended many special events at the nursing facility where he cooks. Standard Buddy fare are petits fours, gourmet cheese and crackers and delicious shellfish, along with ice sculptures on the table. Still, Buddy worries if he is doing what he is called to do. He confided to me one day that he wanted to be closer to God. I was so astonished by his desire, because I see his life as totally intertwined with God. Everything Buddy does is done with such love and tenderness and care. If he isn't of God, no one is. Someone should rearrange the letters on his door some night, so they read DEITARY instead of DIETARY.

Yet Buddy is like all human beings, full of doubt and wondering. He even told me of his recurrent dream in which he finds himself working for much more money in an enormous hotel kitchen. "I wake up so worried, Bethany," Buddy said. "I look around and say 'where are my people? My old people? I can't leave them!'"

And Buddy won't! He's doing what he was meant to do—with extraordinary grace, a gift to all who know him!

 TODAY: Honor the gifts you work with.

Being isolated in a completely self-sufficient environment, your residents can become pretty content with their world. Once they get the hang of the routine, they can find comfort with the familiar.

Repeating the facility's routines every day, staff can become pretty assured too. Not that you let your guard down, but you don't think about crises or emergencies.

When the flood hit the city of Montpelier in March of 1992, nobody had been thinking about how to care for residents in a flood. But the basement at the Gary Home for the Aged did flood, and the ladies who live there had to be transported immediately to a temporary shelter. Quick decisions had to be made, such as what essential items each resident needed, how should careplans and medications be removed, and whether the original patient charts should be removed from the building or copies be made.

Fortunately for all, a happy ending eventually prevailed, and the ladies returned to their dried-out home.

Take a minute today and think about what natural disasters might come your way: tornadoes, hurricanes, fires or even just electrical blackouts. The more staff are able to manage the unexpected, the more calm your residents will remain.

Are you ready for these emergencies? Does your facility's staff need more preparation?

TODAY: Think about handling an emergency.

Talking with our teenagers, it's hard to believe there can be so many misunderstanding when both parties speak English! Communication is truly an art.

At your facility there may well be residents who aren't fluent in English or even used to speaking it. There may be others who can't speak at all, but use some kind of sign language that only their families really understand.

The nursing facility that is truly committed to the well-being of residents will go to great lengths to make communication be the best it can be. That means finding sign language interpreters and even translators for those residents who speak a foreign tongue.

At the nursing facility my grandmother lives in, much of the staff is from Haiti and speaks a French dialect. My grandmother has been frustrated by this situation, as sometimes the staff speak their language in front of her and she can't understand what they are saying.

Making sure that everyone has someone who understands him or her is very important. Those residents who have suffered a stroke or have some other physical disability that alters their speech need special attention too. Find the one staff person who can understand the resident; make sure the two of them can get together daily.

TODAY: Keep communication open.

Do you have the tendency to think that there is an answer for every question you ask, that you just need to ask the right person and you'll learn what you need to know? Did you ever consider the possibility the answer doesn't exist, that it is up to you to discover the answer?

This is particularly true when it comes to techniques for providing care to dementia patients. Some of this land is really uncharted; nobody has been there before. And, like Thomas Edison, you need to invent plenty of answers and solutions in order to settle on one good idea.

At The Arbors, a nursing and assisted living center, the staff has been encouraged to be creative in working with dementia patients. Management knows that the staff are pioneers. After several months of observing and caring for Alzheimer's patients, two aides decided they needed to make a training video on the "do's and don'ts" of caregiving.

The administrator got them a video camera and some video tape and granted some time away from direct caregiving so they could produce the video. After hours of taping and editing, the two women completed a short, powerful training film that has been used in training sessions statewide. This video not only helped staff with some very successful approaches, but it also gave others the idea that they, too, can develop training tools. Why not? You are the people who most understand the circumstances of your patients.

TODAY: What training tools can you design?

Christian literature has many beautiful images of Jesus. None is as powerful for me as that of the shepherd.

No, I have never owned sheep. What I know about them comes from a few visits to a farm, talking to breeders, reading articles. Sheep are extremely useful to the world. At some of the ski resorts in Vermont, sheep graze the trails in the summer, mowing the grass. And of course their fleece is sheared for spinning and their meat sold for eating.

Not violent or moody animals, sheep definitely have made themselves valued members of the farm community.

Still, sheep are not so independent that they don't need a shepherd. In fact they usually need a shepherd who has a crook and a sheep dog. For, as useful as they are, sheep have a tendency to wander and forget what they are about.

Imagining that we are the sheep and our bosses are the shepherds, I like this last fact about sheep—they must be led, not driven. While cattle are driven by cowboys on horseback, usually using whips, sheep only need to have a good shepherd to follow. In fact, they can't be driven.

As you look around your facility, ask yourself, "Am I the kind of worker, the kind of person, that others would want to follow? Could I make a good shepherd?"

TODAY: Be a good sheep and a good shepherd.

Is it just me, or does *The Price is Right* run twenty-four hours a day on a closed-circuit network for nursing facilities? I don't care what time of day or night I drop into a facility, I can hear, "Come on down!" blaring from someone's room.

Like static on the radio, we can get used to annoying background noise. When I mention the racket the television is causing, I'm often met with an almost baffled face. "Oh, I didn't notice," I'm told.

As more and more residents get their own televisions, this problem is compounded. In some homes earphones are becoming more and more common. Hooray! This minor adaptation can make life for everyone much more pleasant.

Americans have come to substitute the television for real conversation. Marshall MacLuan called television "the third parent." In a nursing facility, it could be labeled "an activity aide." All too often residents are parked in front of a television and left for hours.

Some anthropologists believe we are fascinated with the flickering pictures on a television screen because they meet our primordial need to stare at a fire. Perhaps a video of a fireplace or an aquarium would be more appropriate to run on the screen.

TODAY: Don't let TV baby-sit your patients.

Aren't great families great?

Those grown sons who manage on their way home from work to stop and check on dad, maybe even read the paper to him, play a game of cribbage, feed him dinner?

We often dwell on what families don't do and miss the wonderful acts of loving kindness that actually occur, such as the granddaughter who brings a homemade apple pie for the night nurses. And I know of a lady who knits about a hundred pairs of mittens every year for the facility's Christmas bazaar. This lady's mom died years ago at the facility, and she herself has moved to another state. But faithfully, every December, a box of handmade mittens arrives.

Bob volunteers five days a week at the facility his wife died in. Long before her death, Alice had stopped recognizing Bob. But plenty of other residents know and love this gregarious man. Even after Alice died, Bob has kept visiting and volunteering.

Then there is the only child of an Alzheimer's patient living in a nursing facility 800 miles away. Unable to visit his mother more than twice a year, he walked into a nursing facility near his home and said, "I can't visit my mom, so I would like to visit someone else's." What an answer to prayer he's been!

Some family members even have volunteered to testify in the Vermont Legislature, lobbying lawmakers about the importance of fully funding the Medicaid program.

TODAY: Thank the families!

The Bible's long-suffering Job has a contemporary, the lead character J.B. from Archibald MacLeish's play "J.B." J.B. is a successful and climbing businessman who loses everything. His children are killed in horrible accidents; his business fails; bombs fall. Even his wife leaves him and curses God. In the final scene, J.B. and his wife Sarah are reunited as she returns to him. Their home and neighborhood are ashes; the night sky is pitch black.

> J.B.: It's too dark to see.
> She turns, pulls his head down between her hands and kisses him.
> Sarah: Then blow on the coal of the heart, my darling.
> J.B.: The coal of the heart...
> Sarah: It's all the light now.
> Blow on the coal of the heart.
> The candles of the churches are out.
> The lights have gone out of the sky.
> Blow on the coal of the heart
> And we'll see by and by...
> We'll see where we are.
> The wit won't burn and the wet soul smolders.
> Blow on the coal of the heart and we'll know...
> We'll know... (Curtain)

In those moments of incredible sorrow and suffering, when there truly seems to be no hope, help renew hope for one another, staff and residents alike.

TODAY: Blow on the coal of the heart.

Worker injuries in nursing facilities continue to rise. As more and more residents are unrestrained, staff are placed in tougher and tougher situations. Difficult patients hit and attack staff, twisting arms and shoulders. Chairs and other objects are thrown.

Other unsteady patients fall, and staff reach up to break their falls, only to injure themselves.

Plenty of consultants are marketing workshops designed to help your staff learn how to lift, transfer and even to help residents safely use the toilet. Other experts will come and tell you how administrators can reduce claims of injury by using a company doctor, light-duty assignments and more.

But has anyone talked about teaching staff to be more relaxed and at ease with their bodies? How to move more gracefully?

Hannah Dennison, a dancer and dance teacher, has conducted several workshops for nurses' aides on creative movement. Participants sometimes think some of Hannah's exercises are a bit strange, but they help staff loosen up and become comfortable with how they walk, stand and move. Avoiding injury by moving quickly and smoothly is just as important as lifting properly.

Making friends with your physical body and accepting its strengths and weaknesses will help outside the workplace as well.

TODAY: Take a dance class.

It may feel like you work twenty-four hours a day, seven days a week, but, fortunately, you don't.

Still, it seems things happen when you aren't at work, once-in-a-lifetime things that you sure wish you hadn't missed.

Nothing feels so unfair as when one of your favorite patients dies when you're not at work. Walking into his or her room the next day and seeing an empty bed, or, worse still, someone else in the bed, is nothing you want to experience twice. Once is one time too many.

So how can you be at home and at work? You can't. But you can work to develop a system, such as a telephone network, that will alert concerned, but absent, staff to all major changes in residents' conditions.

Interested staff could provide their phone numbers to the office crew or to the director of nursing or to whoever has agreed to head up the information exchange. You could ask to be called when there is a sense that a patient is failing or about to take a change for the worse (or whatever you want to know about, even if her son finally visits!). Once informed, you could then decide if you want to come in or not.

This notification service may seem obvious, but it is not that common. What generally happens is staff find out after the fact, and the loss is three times as hard to accept.

Why not consider helping each other out? The residents will surely benefit too by having their favorite caregiver nearby.

TODAY: Develop a telephone alert system.

Job security. In tough economic times, layoffs are common. "Downsizing" is the nice way to talk about it when companies reduce the size of their staffs, usually squeezing out a lot of middle management.

The good news is, as long as you're a caregiver, you'll never have to worry about having a job. The age group you care for is the fastest growing on earth. In 1990 there were more than 31 million Americans over the age of sixty-five. By the year 2000 there are going to be forty million.

Looking at "older old," the over 85 group, the number is supposed to double between 1990 and the year 2010!

There are about 15,000 nursing homes in the United States, caring for 1.6 million patients. Few new facilities are being built, so as time goes by the competition for these beds will get more intense. And that means the need for your services and skills will be all the more critical.

TODAY: Feel job secure.

October

When I was a kid I sometimes spoke pig Latin with my friend Mary when my brothers were around. We thought we were so clever, keeping the boys out of our secrets. I can also remember how incredibly angry and frustrated the gibberish made my brothers. They hated being left out.

In nursing facilities it is all too easy to talk about patients as if they weren't present. Pig Latin isn't the language, but some healthcare terminology can make things sound pretty foreign and confusing.

Visitors will frequently put staff in this awkward position, saying things like, "Would she like to have some candy?" when the patient is totally capable of describing her needs.

When patients have trouble communicating, it sometimes seems simpler to speak about or for them. Stutterers, stroke patients and others with speech impairments can truly try your patience. Resist filling in the blanks! Permit them the respect and dignity of speaking for themselves. Whenever possible, engage patients in conversations.

TODAY: Talk to, not about, patients.

When Elsie Kerrick turned 105 years of age, she told the staff of McFarland House Nursing Home in Barre that she only wanted one thing: a ride in a hot air balloon.

How many of us would have listened to Elsie and said, "Uh huh. What else do you want, Elsie?" Wouldn't we be tempted to get something easier, less of an outrageous request?

Fortunately for Elsie, the McFarland staff listened intently and took Elsie very seriously. If a hot air balloon ride was what she wanted, they would make it happen.

Such an energy for the unusual reminds me of a prayer written by Sister Ruth Fox, OSB. "May God bless you with the foolishness to think that you can make a difference in this world, so that you will do the things which others tell you can not be done."

Sister Ruth also wrote, "May God bless you with discontent at easy answers, half-truths, superficial relationships, so that you will live from deep within your heart."

Buying Elsie another pair of slippers or a robe was just too easy and superficial. Watching her face go skyward with a glorious grin made everyone know they had done the right thing, that they had made a difference.

TODAY: Be blessed with foolishness.

Everyone who knows us knows only a snapshot of our lives. Our teachers remember one side of us, our first employer another. The memories and opinions of our friends are yet another snapshot. Perhaps no one, other than our spouse or children, knows the full picture. For the residents of nursing facilities, the most that is typically known is the snapshot taken in the last years of life. Staff haven't been through their patients' childbearing or child rearing years. So little of the past is known.

Still, these snapshots in time are precious, if incomplete. When Katherine Taggard died in August of 1992 at eighty-nine, the staff at Thompson House Nursing Home in Brattleboro wrote down some of their fond memories for the facility newsletter:

> A person close to nature, Katherine loved birds, trees, plants and flowers and took enormous care in growing them. Every month she would go out on the patio to experience the full moon.

What a terrific image that paragraph conjures up. How many of us, so wrapped up in the busyness of the day, even notice what phase the moon is in? Katherine kept that link with the heavens, a link that the whole facility enjoyed. Her horizon and world were surprisingly wide, connecting her to mysteries well beyond the four walls of Thompson House. What a fine reminder she was to all that life is bigger than time cards, med charts or incident reports. Life is about the changing seasons, gardens and phases of the moon.

TODAY: Take time to notice the moon.

October 4

A few times I've been visiting a nursing facility after normal business hours and I've needed to make a phone call. During the day, I have always been able to use an office phone. But at night and on weekends I have experienced what staff and residents do when making calls—the lack of privacy.

Perhaps your nursing facility is different, and you have a private, quiet place where you can make calls. If so, consider yourself blessed and among the few who have such grand accommodations. What is more frequently the case is that the pay phone is right smack dab in the middle of everything. Classic pay phone locations are at the entrance, in the lobby, next to the elevator or nurses' station. Not exactly soundproof settings!

Beyond the inconvenience of trying to hear above the noisy environment, callers must share their calls with whomever is around. Other residents, visitors and staff will frequently be entertained by someone else's private call.

Federal laws require that patients have access to phones in private places. Staff deserve the same arrangements. If your facility scores poorly on phone privacy, why not bring up the matter at your next staff meeting? The phone company will usually install phones wherever you ask.

TODAY: Find a private place to install the pay phone.

During times of shortages, human beings tend to hoard. When the US was at war with Germany and Japan in the 1940s, Americans were told they could only have a small amount of sugar stored in their kitchen pantries. To avoid being prosecuted for having an illegal amount of sugar, many women mixed cinnamon with the sugar. Technically they no longer had too much white sugar.

Hoarding wonderful people and stories is a crime many nursing facilities are guilty of, though they aren't knowingly breaking the law. Housed in the facility are dozens of fascinating residents, all with incredibly full, adventurous pasts.

When I was introduced to Winnie, I had no idea this small, compact lady had been a friend of Amelia Earhart. "I used to work for the railroads," Winnie explained. She had gotten her job using the initial "W" instead of "Winnie," and she figured she was hired because the personnel department didn't realize she was a woman. "In those days, trains and airlines were governed by the same department. So, when Amelia came to Vermont, she would always give me a plane ride."

Winnie's stories didn't stop with flight. She also learned to drive a car in a Rolls Royce that had been owned by Winston Churchill. Seems Mrs. Churchill hadn't liked the interior of the Rolls, so it ended up on a used car lot in White River Junction. There, a relative of Winnie's arranged for her to take driving lessons in the Rolls.

Realizing more people would like to hear these stories, I recommended the facility get some students or reporters in to write them down. Talking to Winnie was a lot more fun than reading a textbook.

TODAY: Don't hoard resident stories.

The Army challenges its recruits to "be all that you can be."

Being the "maximum you" involves a lot of elements, including a willingness to remain open and learn new ways. At a nursing facility, dealing with people remains much the same from day to day, but much is changing too.

Learning happens most effortlessly when we are simply watching others go about their business. As an observer, we don't have to defend our way. We can simply consider the new or different approach.

Apprenticeships are founded on this belief that it is by seeing the master in action that the pupil can best learn the skills of a trade. Serving an apprenticeship doesn't mean just learning how to copy or mimic the master. Apprenticing is not limited to becoming a good follower. Instead, being an apprentice means the student fully intends to become as expert as his teacher, to become a master himself.

Aristotle said it was greater to be a master craftsman than simply an artisan, because the master knows not only how to do things, but why they are done.

In eastern religions, the guru is the master that people apprentice to. Quite literally, the Hindi meaning of the word "guru" is the two words "gu," meaning dark, and "ru," meaning light. The spiritual leader brings his people from dark to light.

Look around the facility. Who can you apprentice under? Who can teach you about care and life? Who could be your guru?

 TODAY: Find a guru; be a guru.

Okay, okay. So Mary makes the best corners when changing the sheets on the bed, and Sal does the cutest French braids.

But what about hidden talents? What can your staff and residents do as stars in a talent show?

I once saw a nursing facility performance of a Hee Haw show. Even the residents were blowing into old whiskey jugs, with others playing the washboards.

Who can yodel? Tap dance? Square dance? Sing? Tell jokes? Do aerobic dance? How about a skit about life in the kitchen, or based on other behind-the-scenes stories?

Nothing is more fun than poking fun at each other. Why not organize a talent show complete with master of ceremonies and popcorn sales? Have some fun!

TODAY: Time for a talent show!

I just heard about a married couple's fight involving two people who have been together almost a decade. Seems he didn't like the incense she burned, so he poured aftershave all over the rug. These are adults, too!

The point is, neither our age nor our relationship make us immune from roommate hassles. People get on people's nerves. And when an older person is forced to share a room with a stranger, is it any surprise problems arise?

Listening to complaints with compassion and attention, without taking sides or getting emotionally involved—that's an art. After all, if your patients can't talk to you, whom can they tell?

My own grandmother had three roommates for a while, but actually managed to maintain control over everything important, such as the television, because she was the only one of the quartet who was not demented. When a new, alert roommate moved in, the TV battle began. A creative staff person resolved the conflict by getting the roommate earphones to listen to the TV so my grandmother wouldn't be bugged.

Another creative arrangement I saw involved a totally deaf resident and another who moaned twenty-four hours a day. Paired up, neither of them complained about the other.

Nursing facilities are always asking people to compromise or follow the program in the name of a smooth operation. The more we can creatively accommodate our residents, the more at home and at peace they will feel.

 TODAY: Handle hassles creatively.

Frances is a hardworking, considerate soul. You will never hear Frances run anybody down or whine. She is like the little engine that could, chugging along, pulling her share of the load.

One of the special treats Frances enjoys is being a bit spoiled by a few of her patients. These folks know a heart of gold when they see it, and they clearly want to be kind to Frances.

Working the night shift, Frances is a busy aide, running around the wing, getting everyone ready for bed. At Josie's room, the scene is always the same. Josie has saved some part of one of her meals that day: a cup of pudding, a cookie, some chips. Frances enters Josie's room, and Josie always says the same thing, "Hi, Frances, your lunch is on the little table by the door."

Frances then looks over and sees her goodie sitting on a napkin. "Oh, thank you, Josie," she beams, "You are so good to me! It will be nice to have with my coffee tonight. You've made my night."

Frances and Josie take care of each other. Nothing fancy, nothing complicated, no money is exchanged. They are just friends.

TODAY: Be good to one another.

Everyone asks Gary and Alicia Marcotte the same question: "Why llamas?"

And to everyone who asks, the Marcottes give the same answer, "Why not?"

At Maple Lane, their beautiful nursing facility nestled in the rolling countryside of Vermont, two llamas roam the huge fenced-in grounds. The year-old animals, Beckett and Prince Valiant, are gentle, intelligent and fascinating. Residents of the nursing facility and assisted living facility get a big kick out of watching the llamas. Even more interested in these two creatures, which look like goats that married camels, are the children at the facility day care. How lucky can kids get? They get to come to work with their parents, have their choice of adopted grandparents and laps, and pet llamas.

As Gary wrote in the Maple Lane newsletter, "Llamas give llots of llove." With such a pedigree, of course they belong at a nursing facility!

TODAY: Why not a llama?

In college I met a woman named Yvonne who had lived most of her life in a wheelchair. Having contracted polio as a child, she was also dependent on a ventilator.

One afternoon we were talking about "what if."

"What if you could walk and move your arms for one day, Yvonne. What would you do?" I asked.

Yvonne surprised me. I expected to hear about swimming and bike riding and dancing and piano playing.

"I would punch everyone in the nose who has patted me on the head all these years," she said with defiance.

Being short because she sat in a wheelchair, Yvonne felt she was often treated as a child or a cute non-adult. I have never forgotten her words or her angry face that afternoon.

In most nursing homes most residents are confined to wheelchairs. Do they experience what Yvonne so disliked? A few newer facilities have actually designed their nurses' stations to be low desks so the nurse sits at eye level with the person in a wheelchair. What a difference this must make in conversations and feelings of dependence! Adapting a facility to wheelchair height can be as extensive as energy and budget permit. Some homes have elevated outdoor gardens so their residents can weed and tend to plants from a seated position; others have aquariums set up at just the right height.

TODAY: Is your home wheelchair-friendly?

Poor Bonnie. She had become so uncertain of herself, of her value as a nurse. A lovely, slender, kind woman with a true sparkle in her eye, Bonnie had spent many years operating a children's day-care with her sister. When the time came to make a career change, she decided to work in a residential care home for older women.

An idea person who enjoyed creating programs and activities, Bonnie brought her enthusiasm for crafts and group events to the facility. After all, she had always had a million projects going for the kids; why would she stop now?

At first the ladies did not know what to do with Bonnie's cheerful questions: "What would you like to do? Where would you like to go on a drive? Who would you like to have come and visit?" No one had ever asked these questions. B.B. (Before Bonnie) life had consisted of meals, baths and the occasional trip to the doctor's office.

As time progressed the residents began to answer Bonnie's questions. A fall foliage car ride was planned, including a stop for ice tea at Bonnie's home in the country. A tour of a famous ice cream company, Ben and Jerry's, was arranged.

Quite abruptly one day the head nurse called Bonnie to her office for a conference. "I am not at all pleased with how you are fitting in here," said the head nurse gruffly. "You are just too enthusiastic, and the others don't like working with you."

Too enthusiastic? Bonnie kept repeating the phrase in her head all that week, worrying that she was, in some way, making life worse for the residents. Looking objectively at the residents, they seemed to be thrilled with Bonnie's approach to work. After talking with friends who cared about her, Bonnie came to see the problem wasn't herself or her enthusiasm. The problem was the unhappy, burned-out staff.

TODAY: Welcome enthusiastic staffers.

In the movie *Oh, God, Book II*, the character Tracy has a conversation with God about why bad things happen. God tells Tracy sometimes there is a purpose for things that we aren't aware of.

God: I know this sounds like a cop-out, but there's really nothing I can do about pain and suffering. It's built into the system.

Tracy: Which you invented.

God: Right. But my problem is I never could figure out how to make anything with just one side to it.

Tracy: One side?

God: Did you ever see a front without a back?

Tracy: No.

God: A top without a bottom?

Tracy: No.

God: An up without a down?

Tracy: No.

God: Okay. And there can't be good without bad. Life without death. Pleasure without pain. That's how it is. If I take sad away, happy has to go with it. If anyone knows another way, I'd wish they'd put it in the suggestion box.

In your nursing facility, you see plenty of both sides of life. Sometimes you seem to see a lot of pain and suffering. As if your patients aren't coping with enough loss and sorrow, they must be told that a favorite grandchild has just been diagnosed with cancer, or a son has died in a car accident, or a daughter is getting a divorce. Sometimes, it seems like more than the dear old soul can bear.

When bad news must be delivered, make sure the staffer closest to the resident is working and nearby. Such moments call for an abundance of tenderness and compassion.

TODAY: Break bad news with love.

Any occasion is a fine time for music. The next time the spirit moves you, perhaps before a meal, why not teach everyone the following version of "Bless this House." Thanks to the National Council on Aging's Interfaith Coalition for providing the lyrics.

Just ask someone in the office to make copies of the words and, if possible, enlarge them so your residents can more easily follow along.

BLESS THE OLD

Bless the old, O Lord, we pray.
Keep them safe by night and day.
Bless the feet that never cease
walking on the path of peace.
Bless the touch of older hands
Showing someone understands!
Bless their hearts, that they may prove
Ever open to joy and love!
Bless the visions of their eyes
Handed on to make us wise.
Bless the ears attuned to hear
Hopefulness in each new year.
Bless the lips that move to raise
Songs of majesty and praise.
Bless the goodness they have known.
Bless the ways that they have grown.
Bless us all, that ever we
May trust, O Lord, in Thee!

TODAY: Sing a blessing.

What do your friends know about your work?

"Well, I know she gets her hands into some pretty awful situations."

"She doesn't get paid enough."

"Some of the people she works with are really lazy."

Just what are the messages we give our families and friends about work? Would anyone ever want to come and work with us, given what they've heard?

While life does include some pretty rotten situations, every day has its high points and sunny moments too. We need to remember to share these precious stories with those who are close to us.

If life is what we make it, we need to watch what we say and believe about our place of work. Most of our waking day is spent in the facility. Let's pledge to pass along the good news. Make sure your friends hear about the lovely patients you are privileged to care for, and about those coworkers who make your day so good.

TODAY: Tell the good news.

In our more disparaging moments, we call them Mutt and Jeff. You know who I'm referring to—those odd couples that seem to get paired up in a facility.

Sometimes a man and a woman; more often two women together. One of them is usually in an early stage of dementia, pretty confused about who and where she is. Somehow the more domineering, clear thinking one adopts her, and away they go.

Usually you see them walking the halls, stopping in the activities room, the living room, or anywhere there is a crowd. Not staying long, the strong one orders the frailer one to "come along," and the wandering continues.

Such liaisons are most often harmless—no one is being victimized. Rarely, the weaker of the two can be taken advantage of or bullied. Keep your eyes and ears open for any verbal abuse. No one deserves to be pushed around, especially when they are in your facility to be protected and pampered.

TODAY: Monitor partnerships.

October 17

One of your worst nightmares is the patient who will not change her clothes. You try every trick in the book—all the techniques you've used with your own kids, and then some. But forget it; she won't get out of those clothes.

Up to a point, such independence deserves your respect. Many people have grown up in cultures or families where frequent changes of outfits are considered strange. So you go with the flow, trying to replace a shirt or sweater whenever you can.

But there does come a point when not only personal hygiene but the personal space of other patients becomes a concern. No one should have to share a dinner table or bingo game with someone who smells bad because they haven't changed.

It seems patients suffering with dementia are most frequently the folks who refuse to get undressed. Because reason doesn't work, creative and compassionate staff need to try other mechanisms.

One of the most successful tricks, when done very carefully, involves the "oops I'm a klutz" accident. The primary aide who is most trusted by the resident "by accident" spills a small amount of warm water on the patients pants or sleeve.

"Oh, what a klutz I am!" the staffer cries. "Let's get you out of these wet clothes."

This works quite often, and even allows the resident to reassure the employee and show some consideration.

TODAY: Help patients wear clean clothes.

I was delivering something to the activities department.

Waiting for Sandy, the director, I began to visit with a stooped little lady curled up in her wheelchair like a shrimp. I think she knew me as the woman who occasionally led the Friday morning worship service. I later learned her name was Ilene.

"I bet you wonder why I married Mr. Johnson," she said.

I looked at her and said I hadn't known she was married, but would she like to tell me about it? I was unprepared for what became a kind of confession.

"My friend died on the kitchen floor," Ilene said. "She had asked me to help her abort the baby. She couldn't have another. She bled to death. I promised her I would marry her husband and raise her kids."

Not even forty words, and Ilene's guilt and pain tumbled out into the day. I listened, never moving, giving Ilene the time and attention she needed.

"Have you forgiven yourself, Ilene?"

"No," said Ilene, unable to look me in the eye.

"God has forgiven you, Ilene. A long time ago," I said forcefully. "You helped your friend because you loved her. And you kept your promise. It is time you forgave youself."

Ilene sighed and started to cry. I wheeled her to her room, where she asked for help using the toilet.

Less than a month later I read Ilene's obituary. I believe she had forgiven herself.

TODAY: Listen to your patient's fears.

October 19

We all bring who we are to our jobs. If you were raised to always be kind to strangers, you're probably saying hello all day long to people who pass in the hall. If you were told never to pry into others' lives, you most likely never ask a personal question of anyone.

Some people find the presence of cultural quirks and habits inappropriate for the workplace. "Everybody should dress and act the same, like professionals," some managers will say. "Keep your way of doing things out of the picture."

Such an attitude is pretty doomed, though, because employees can't stop being themselves just because they are in the nursing home. If they've always whistled while they've worked, they'll keep whistling.

At one prestigious home for retired Jewish ladies, the administration went to great lengths to maintain the familiar customs associated with meals and holidays. As much as possible, patterns of the Jewish culture were followed.

But no Jewish women applied to work at the home. Instead, the direct care staff was almost exclusively black women from the inner city. These caregivers brought their culture with them, which included braiding the long white hair of their Jewish patients into intricate and often colorful corn rows!

At first, management flipped their wigs (pardon the pun). The coiffures made the director of nursing's hair stand on end (pardon the pun again). But gradually, seeing how the residents got a kick out of their new hairstyles, everyone relaxed. It was fun to try a different 'do!

TODAY: Bring your culture to work.

Claire was more than unusual. She was a one-of-a-kind, eccentric character, the perfect spirit to work as an activities director.

No one ever could predict Claire or her plans. Her ideas seemed to come from a bottomless well of creative juices, a well found on a faraway planet full of wild and wonderful fantasies.

One summer night, Claire announced she was taking a carload of adventurous residents camping. "I know an abandoned house on a friend's farm. We're going to sleep there," she said with excitement. "Grab your pillows, lots of blankets and some toilet paper. We're out of here!"

Such excursions are the stuff that administrators have nightmares over. I'm quite certain that Claire's boss's first words the next morning were, "Pass the Pepto, please!" I'm also quite certain that the words first uttered by the campers went something like this: "Wow! We are really alive! We did something crazy and amazing. Thanks, Claire!"

TODAY: Be unpredictable.

Caring for other people can be dangerous work. Look at the injuries around you, the elastic bandages on wrists, ankles, knees. When people are confused because of dementia, they are easily upset. Not understanding why you are undressing them, or helping them from one room to another, patients panic and strike out.

No caregiver needs to take such behavior personally. If your patient was oriented to his or her situation, he or she wouldn't be hitting anyone. Be compassionate and empathetic.

Beyond responding with our hearts, smart caregivers also need to learn about how to protect themselves from injury. At Cedar Hill in Windsor, the local police force has provided staff with free in-services on Akido, a martial art. No, aides aren't being taught how to deliver a karate chop to their patients! Yes, they are getting instructions on how to use peaceful resistance and other techniques to diffuse physical attacks.

Staff at Cedar Hill report a dramatic reduction in such incidents and injuries since the Akido training.

TODAY: Protect yourself and prevent injuries.

The days race by in a nursing home. One day there are two residents in 236; the next day there is one resident and one empty bed. Usually operating with a waiting list, most facilities quickly fill the bed.

Whenever possible it is much healthier for all involved if the bed can remain open for at least twenty-four hours. This waiting time provides staff and residents with an opportunity to absorb the loss, to deal with the death, to begin to move on.

At Greensboro Nursing Home, the certified nurses' aides contribute money at the beginning of the year to their Flower Fund. When a death occurs, money in the Flower Fund is used to buy a rose which is placed on the empty bed.

The flower remains on the bed until a new resident moves in. For the residents who continue to live at the facility, it is very comforting to wheel or walk past the room and see the rose on the bed. They all know that when their day comes they will not be forgotten. The flower memorial has a powerful, positive effect on everyone.

TODAY: Start a flower fund.

Convenience can be a wicked thing.

Television is a convenient baby-sitter for children, but aren't hours and hours of daily viewing damaging?

Eating at fast-food restaurants every night is easy, but does the body not suffer being deprived of fresh fruit and vegetables?

In nursing facilities, standard nursing practice has traditionally involved plenty of behavior-altering medications and manual restraints. Chemical and physical restraints have been given many sorts of labels, but basically they are tools of convenience. Isn't it easier to care for a wing of thirty patients when the wanderers are tied in their chairs? Isn't it easier to tend thirty noisy patients when the most belligerent are snowed under?

But, quite frankly, who ever said nursing policies should be based on what is most convenient for staff? In fact, isn't the patient's welfare the key factor when establishing standards of care? So the staff is inconvenienced! They are, after all, being paid to work. The residents, however, are paying for care.

TODAY: Make no care policies for staff convenience.

When I hear stories of creative staff caring for challenging residents, I end up by saying, "I can't decide who is the most amazing, staff or patients."

When Hattie insisted on working as a hostess at all facility meals, the staff was caught off guard. This was one situation they hadn't run into. It seems Hattie had worked most of her life as a hostess in a large hotel dining room. Her talent was in seating people graciously, periodically checking on them and assuring them, "Your waitress will be right with you."

Finding herself in a large dining room, Hattie felt completely at home and would seat her fellow residents throughout the entire meal, never even considering the idea of sitting and eating herself. "Now?" she would say incredulously. "I'm working!"

After a short staff meeting, her primary caregivers decided they had to make sure Hattie ate first every day, before anyone else was served. Indeed this solution was precisely what Hattie was accustomed to. Seated near the kitchen door, Hattie would enjoy her quick meal and then get ready for the onslaught of guests.

TODAY: Do what works.

At first the staff thought any kind of memorial for residents who died at the facility would be considered morbid.

"I don't think the other residents will like hearing about dead people," said the activities director.

"Do you think they don't know they're going to die?" another staffer asked.

"No, but this seems so, so . . ." The activities director's voice trailed off. She was uncomfortable talking about death and believed the residents felt the same way.

A few months later, after some death and dying in-services were conducted at the facility, the idea of a wall memorial was discussed again. This time the activities director was interested, even excited, about the possibility.

"I think we could do something really beautiful," she said.

The staff agreed on holding memorial services twice a year. In the activities program, patients now make ceramic angels using the facility kiln. When someone dies, an angel is given to the family at a memorial service.

TODAY: Give away angels.

Why is it that so many caregivers are battered women? What is it in the gentle, caring nature of nurses' aides and nurses that makes them prey to brutal men?

When the story first hit the news that fall day, no one could believe it was true. A twenty-one-year-old cook at a nursing facility had been dragged out of the building at gun point by her estranged husband. After a two day search, the two were found dead in their car. First he shot her, then himself. They left a young son.

For the staff who witnessed the violent abduction, the incident was the most upsetting experience of their lives. Diane had been with them working in the kitchen one minute and, the next minute, she was gone. They had felt powerless.

Diane's husband had made a reputation for himself the whole year, as she would come to work bruised and injured. Finally she had gotten a restraining order and he had moved out. But the beatings continued.

Following Diane's death, the facility began to hold support group meetings for battered women and to seek professional help for their staff. A petition was circulated to collect signatures calling for stricter laws for abusers. Staff delivered the petition to the state legislature the following session. The whole facility became sadder and wiser overnight as the abuse came out of the closet.

TODAY: Stop abuse.

Many of us think the best way to handle pain or sadness is to keep it to ourselves. "What's the point of sharing?" we wonder, not wanting to burden our friends or family.

Lola hadn't been one to blurt her feelings out to just anyone. In fact, since her mother had died, she didn't tell anyone much of anything. Most of the time she could swallow her suffering, put on her uniform and go to work. She almost always felt better just getting into her nurses' aide routine; it helped her forget her troubles.

On this day, though, she couldn't contain her grief. Her son was getting another divorce, his third, this time leaving two more children. His alcoholism was destroying the lives of everyone around her, and he would listen to no one.

When she saw the old priest leave a resident's room that morning, Lola lost it. "Father, I need to talk," she said quickly.

The priest found a quiet corner in an unoccupied sun room. "What is it, my dear?"

Lola spilled out her story and her tears. The words tumbled; her shoulders shook. The priest nodded and would only say "continue" or "and what else, dear?"

After about twenty minutes, Lola's body relaxed and she stopped crying. "Oh, Father," she said, "Thank you so much for this great talk. I can't tell you how much better I feel. I should have come to you a long time ago. Thank you so much."

The priest gave her a loving hug, and they said goodbye.

Sharing our grief is like pouring our cup into the great pot called humanity. When we spill our pain, it is diluted by others, and we begin to feel we can move forward. Lola's situation is a perfect example of this shared and thus diluted pain. In fact the priest never said anything; he just listened, as Lola emptied herself.

TODAY: Be ready to listen and to share.

The arts and health care make terrific partners. So much of music, drama and poetry is based on poignant stories of life—birth, death, relationships.

Being wrapped up in our work, it is not surprising that we do not always see the beauty or the preciousness around us.

Bringing a photographer or a painter or even a poet into the facility can totally change the way staff and residents begin to look at their situation. The facility becomes a great stage, a watercolor painting, a living work of art. The faces and hands of your residents are so full of stories—the wrinkles, the knobby knuckles, the missing fingers!

Pictures are worth even more than a thousand words in a nursing facility. One clear black and white photo can tell us more than a short story about the resident and her caregiver.

Wouldn't it be fun to publish a yearbook or a calendar about your facility? Schools do such projects, and everyone loves to buy a copy. Resident and staff poems and pictures could be included in the finished product. Imagine the family members who would like to buy a copy. Think, too, of the fun of creating this project together, to tell the wonderful story of your home.

TODAY: Invite a photographer to come by.

I remember my first ride in a powerboat. It was so exciting. We had brought a cooler with all kinds of soda, a picnic basket full of treats and our fishing poles. A guest of a friend's family, I couldn't believe my good fortune. This was going to be a great day!

About two hours into the ride, I needed to pee. Badly. I was probably ten years old and pretty modest about telling other people when I needed to go to the bathroom. All the free soda! What could I do? I was at their mercy and too shy to tell anyone, too embarrassed.

When we finally stopped at a little island, I had to go so fiercely I couldn't even go! It took me forever in the bushes to relax enough. My memories of that powerboat ride over the years have slipped away; only the need to pee remains clear. My preoccupation with my bodily functions totally dominated the day and my memories of it.

This painful recollection is one I compare to the lives of many nursing facility residents. Confined to a wheelchair, many of them are dependent on others to help them use the toilet. I've visited facilities where residents call and call for help to use the toilet, some near tears. I've noticed that the loud, obnoxious residents often get taken care of first. Is that the behavior required to get our attention?

Despite our busyness, it is of the highest importance that we make sure all residents are toileted when they need to be. Any other standard of care is unacceptable. No one ought to be at someone else's mercy for this most basic bodily need.

 TODAY: Get folks to the toilet on time.

Our splintered world is a constant reminder of just how hard it is for human beings to get along.

Men hurt women; adults hurt children; blacks and whites tangle. The former Soviet Union has become a battle field, as have other major parts of the world.

In your role as a caregiver, your life is about harmony, about getting along, about working out differences.

Poet and playwright Judy Chicago wrote an untitled poem for The Dinner Party about how life might be someday. Listen to the peaceful, cooperative spirit Chicago envisions. See how you are already building such a world:

Then all that has divided us will merge
And then compassion will be wedded to power
And then softness will come to a world that is
harsh and unkind
And then both men and women will be gentle
And then both men and women will be strong
And then no person will be subject to another's
will
And then all will be rich and free and varied
And then the greed of some will give way to the
needs of many
And then all will share equally in the Earth's
abundance
And then all will care for the sick and the weak
and the old
And then all will nourish the young
And then all will cherish life's creatures
And then all will live in harmony with each other
and the Earth
And then everywhere will be called Eden once
again.

TODAY: Practice peace.

Ghosts aren't the only evils lurking on Halloween. These days, children have to beware of the very treats people hand out at the door: Are the cookies poisoned? Do the apples conceal pins or razor blades?

Given this sick turn of events, many parents don't permit their children to trick-or-treat. The custom has become too dangerous, not worth the risk. Missing out on the excitement of Halloween seems so sad though, doesn't it? Your residents can tell wonderful stories of how they or their children would receive delicious homemade caramel apples and popcorn balls on this special night. Why not have your nursing facility become a trick-or-treat center?

Many facilities are providing this service to the children of their community, and it is impossible to determine who benefits the most. The kids get a safe, fun environment to parade their costumes and collect wonderful goodies. The residents have happy disguised youngsters dropping by for a visit. Some facilities even create haunted houses in one room or wing, which adds to the evening's excitement.

Talk the idea over with residents. Open your Halloween House tonight!

TODAY: Invite trick-or-treaters in.

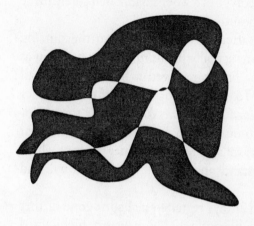

Remember Frank, the turkey hunter you met on June 30? "A man's man" was his description, a rugged individual who had worked a lifetime building roads and bridges.

Learning that Frank was a philosophy student didn't fit the stereotype of a woodsman, but it surely made him a more beautiful person.

Not long after he was admitted to the nursing home (this was actually his third nursing home in as many years), Frank received a book in the mail addressed "To Frank English, student number 32881." *Entitled Philosophies Men Live By,* the author (Davison) promised to "make the insights of the great philosophers available to the beginner in terms which he can understand, and in a fashion which he will find appealing."

Frank had always regretted he hadn't gone further in school. He diligently read his new text, highlighted some sections and underlined others. Tests came and went through the mail, revealing the great determination and mind of student 32881.

Growing more limited in his physical abilities every day, Frank grew more expansive mentally.

"I'm not saying I've gotten soft and believe in God now," Frank said one day when asked about his interest in philosophy. "It's just something I've always wondered about."

TODAY: Avoid stereotyping.

At a self-esteem workshop for nurses' aides, participants were handed a sheet of stationery and a stamped envelope.

"Today," the leader said, "you have been reminded of your worth and value, to yourself and to the people in your care. Now is the time to write yourself a little letter mentioning the important things you have learned. We'll mail it to you in six months when you need to recharge your batteries."

Susan sat for a minute, thinking. "Kind of silly to write myself a letter," she thought, "but I did get a lot out of this program."

Six months later, when Susan's mood had hit a low point and she found herself questioning why she was still at the nursing home, the letter arrived. Opening it, she smiled to herself, pleased she had cared enough about Susan to write.

Dear Susan:

You've come a long way, but you have much further to go. You have to stop feeling that you aren't happy if you can't do everything for everyone. What you do counts for something. If every day you do what you can, the best you can, then it doesn't matter if you've accomplished everything you've set out to do that day.

Be happy with who you are and feel good about what you do. If you love yourself, you can love other people. Smile!

TODAY: Remind yourself of your worth.

When we human beings want to avoid something, we are brilliant. Excuses flow like Niagara Falls; distractions are as common as flies. How many times have you heard the friends and family members of your patients say, "I've been meaning to come over to the nursing home and visit, but I just haven't had the time"? The truth is, walking into a nursing home can be tough.

One small community facility found a way to actually attract visitors, even strangers, into their building. Not only are folks comfortable dropping by; they make a point of it!

Why? Because the rural home started a small bakery, open to the community, and now sells helium-filled balloons for special occasions too. These two features have transformed the facility from a place of dread to a lively center of activity and fun. Local families come by regularly now to pick up bread or cookies. Bouquets of balloons are frequently seen coming through the front door with several beaming children attached.

Not only have these two services made the nursing facility a more "visitor friendly" site, they have made life more interesting for the many residents who spend hours in the front lobby. The world has gotten busier and more stimulating to watch, with a variety of guests to chat with for a while.

TODAY: Can you add a community service?

"I hate politics and I hate the news!" Linda said firmly. While a few staff members were talking about the fighting they had seen on the news last night, Linda wanted no part. "We can't make a difference anyway; nobody can."

Linda is not alone in feeling powerless. When she finally lays down at night, Linda doesn't care about international affairs or the Congress. She just worries because her weekly take-home of less than $200 doesn't pay the bills.

The truth is, paying a little bit of attention to politics can make a big difference. Did you know that the Pentagon, headquarters for America's military efforts, spends $700,000 a minute? That's your tax dollars at work. Still don't care? Do you realize that 7 1/2 minutes worth of Pentagon money would pay you $100 an hour for 25 years?

Maybe it's time we all started to care a little bit about politics and the news. Next time there is an election, make sure everyone in the facility, staff and residents, are registered to vote. Appoint someone to get absentee ballots for the people who can't get to the polling places. (Some nursing homes in Maine have had their facilities declared a polling place!)

Invite politicians to come and tour your facility. Have them work half a day by your side, learning what you do for your wages. See if you can shake a little of that Pentagon change into your pocket. As Buckminster Fuller wrote, do we want money spent on "weaponry or livingry?"

TODAY: Pay attention to politics.

You're already five minutes late leaving for work and now you can't find your keys. G-r-r-r-r. Is there any feeling more aggravating, more annoying?

Imagine facing such a loss of personal property and being too weak or frail to look for the item? That's how your patients feel, sometimes several times a day.

Between the three shifts of staff and the wandering patients, it's no wonder that pocketbooks, glasses, brushes and combs disappear regularly. The less alert patients may not notice what's missing. But those who are still mentally sharp can face incredible frustration whenever something vanishes.

Such occurrences can become so commonplace for us staff that we lose our compassion for the resident who has been ripped off. Instead of comforting them on their loss, and sharing their anger, we get annoyed with their complaining and snap at the victim. Words like, "I know your pocketbook is missing! We're looking for it, okay?" can jump out of our mouths without thought.

When a man or woman's life has been reduced to one half of one small room, whatever personal possessions they still have must be very precious. Let's remember the importance of protecting patients from thefts; when such unfortunate incidents occur, let's be a source of calm, not anxiety.

TODAY: Respect personal property.

In many states, this week is election week. Every four years we elect our president and some members of Congress. During the years in between, a variety of state and local elections are held.

Do you have any former elected officials living in your facility? Town clerks? Justices of the Peace? Former members of your state's house of representatives or senate? Depending on their willingness, it might be great fun to gather these folks together for an informal program. What were the issues they campaigned on? How much money did they spend on a campaign? What was the worst part of running for office?

Other residents who hear the program might enjoy talking about the first time they voted and how many presidential elections they have voted in. Did any of them ever see a US President in person? Who and where?

The day-to-day routine of life in a nursing facility can sometimes drown out what's going on in the world. Who wants to talk about taking medicine and staying dry all day? Don't forget to talk about the world outside the nursing home.

TODAY: Talk about voting.

New staff often find themselves uncomfortable, even repelled, by patients with severe physical disabilities and deformities. The uncommon, sometimes bizarre, look of accident victims makes it difficult to talk to them, let alone to touch them.

Alan Cohen, in his 1983 book called *Rising In Love*, writes of this very experience.

> Mrs. Jorgensen was an elderly woman I met in a nursing home. She was very old, she had no legs or teeth, her eyes were bloodshot, and she involuntarily stuck her tongue out and in every few seconds. The first time I saw her I was very uneasy about her appearance; I gave her a polite smile and stepped past her as quickly as I could. I just didn't want to face her....One day after about six months of seeing Mrs. Jorgensen, as I was walking out of her room I realized I had not been at all conscious of her physical features. I had learned to look past her body and into her soul. And what a beautiful soul it was! She had such a lovely smile, always gave a kind word, and when it came time for exercise class, she tried and worked so hard, bending over in her wheelchair to touch the feet she didn't have. Saints, I discovered, are not confined to cloisters and pilgrimages; they live among us, humbly shining the light of love to ease the burdens of those around them. Mrs. Jorgensen was one of these.

Look for the truly beautiful people in your midst. Tell them they are beautiful.

TODAY: See saints.

As in any big business, so too in a nursing home, the right hand doesn't always know what the left hand is doing. Even in our own families we can wind up with no milk or two gallons of it, depending on who forgot and who remembered to buy some.

The maintenance department has decided today is the day to strip the hall floors. The activities director has a tour of school children walking through any minute.

At one nursing facility, the ordering of supplies was done by two staffers. Nursing supplies were handled by the director of nursing; cleaning supplies where ordered by the director of buildings and grounds. This two-person responsibility would have proved fatal except for the keen eye of a caregiver.

It seems the director of nursing decided each patient should have a bottle of mouthwash, the idea being to prevent germs from being transferred between patients on a shared bottle of mouthwash. The director of buildings and grounds made a similar decision—each bedroom should have its own bottle of window cleaner so staff wouldn't be wasting time carrying or looking for supplies.

The problem? The bottles were the same size, unlabeled, and contained liquid that was almost exactly the same color blue! Yikes! Very fortunately, an alert nurse noticed the similarity, realized the potential for poisoning, and told the administrator immediately. A potential disaster was avoided.

TODAY: Pay attention.

Ever feel embarrassed standing where you are? Parked in front of an "Adults Only" movie theater when we run into an old family friend, we can't wait to mention that we are late for a hair appointment, and this is the only parking spot we could find. We want people to think the best of us, to not write us off.

Residents of nursing facilities who are mentally alert fight this battle daily. Fearing they are being judged in a kind of guilt-by-association, many seem eager to point out, to all visitors and staff, "I have my mind; I'm not like her."

At first these whispered confessions seem silly and out of place. "Why is she telling me that?" the listener wonders. Upon reflecting on the message, one realizes the alert patient doesn't want to be ignored or written off. "Notice me! Talk to me! Treat me like an adult, like your equal!" That is what they are really saying.

With an identity that has been shrinking ever since she moved into your facility, the competent resident is clinging to what she still prizes—her mind. Witnessing so many of her peers with little or no mental strengths, she becomes all the more determined to accent the positive. She isn't criticizing the demented and senile; she is just so glad to not be among them.

TODAY: Engage in an intellectual conversation with a patient.

Like a bottle that washes up on shore with a message from a distant land, your patients arrive at the facility with full lives. Many have been facing the great losses that brought them to your door.

In her moving monologue entitled "Moving On," chaplain Barbara Watts of Birmingham, Alabama, writes of the real life transitions that led one older woman to decide to move to the nursing home. The piece includes twelve separate short conversations between a husband and wife, their children, and, eventually, the widow's thoughts alone. It begins:

> Setting: Mary has sold her home after the death of her husband Joe. It is moving-day and she wanders through the rooms hearing voices, smelling smells, seeing images of the past.
>
> Where do the days go?
> Yesterday this house was alive with sounds and smells.
> The sounds of a husband and wife.
> The sounds of lovemaking.
> "Joe, remember to take the garbage out."
> "Remember to take my pants to the cleaners, Hon."
> "Sometimes you REALLY make me angry."
> "Well, you don't have a corner on that market, DEAR!"
> "I love you."
> "The children are driving me crazy."
> "I've had a hard day at work."
> "Time for dinner, please come on."
> "Just a minute, we're coming."

"How can we afford another child?"
"I hear the baby crying. It's your turn to get up."

Sounds like your house, too? Your patients are full of memories, of pain and joy.

TODAY: Listen to memories.

Martin was a working man. During the hardest working years of his life he worked in a cedar post mill from 4 a.m. till noon every day—then went on to a second job.

His hands told the story. Huge, rough, bent, they had earned many a paycheck.

Part of Martin's daily routine was enjoying the lunch and thermos of coffee his wife packed at 3:30 a.m. Full of leftovers from the night before, the lunch reminded him of the woman he was supporting, the family he was raising.

These days Martin's mind is full of confusion. One of the millions suffering from Alzheimer's disease, Martin wanders about the nursing home looking lost and preoccupied. No longer able to burn his energy doing physical labor, he paces for hours at a time.

Hearing of Martin's lifework from one of his daughters who visited, the nursing home staff made a special lunch arrangement. From that day forward, Martin's noon meal was served out of a lunch box, his coffee in a steel-gray thermos. With the familiar, comforting lunch box and thermos before him, Martin sat contentedly at lunch, a moment of rest in his otherwise restless day.

TODAY: Bring rest to the restless.

Seeing the smiling faces of third-world children kicking an old rusty can down the alleyway reminds us that life is what we make it. Instead of complaining about not having a ball and bat, these poor children find joy. As the saying goes, if you are given a lemon, make lemonade.

Famous playwright George Bernard Shaw wrote:

> I want to be thoroughly used up when I die, for the harder I work the more I live. I rejoice in life for its own sake. Life is no brief candle to me. It is a sort of splendid torch which I have got hold of for the moment, and I want to make it burn as brightly as possible before handing it on to future generations.

On our best days, when we are feeling full of possibility and self-confidence, we all would probably say we want to be thoroughly used up when we die.

But for those prisoners of mental illnesses, life can feel like a cruel torture, an unending sentence of sadness. Many of the people you take care of probably have a diagnosis that includes dementia or senility. How can they rejoice in life?

The staff estimates that Martin, whom you met yesterday, walks ten miles a day through the corridors of the facility, back and forth, round and around. This ritual is his only occupation these days, and he does it with determination. Nothing stops Martin; he is like the mailman in a storm.

The staff have come to celebrate this achievement for Martin, making sure he has comfortable walking shoes and gets offered water and the use of a toilet frequently. They are his support team, helping him "burn as brightly as possible."

TODAY: Support others.

∞

Ben had been a salesman, a man who enjoyed his expense account and his meals on the road. But those days were long over. A series of strokes had left Ben in a wheelchair in a large, four-story nursing home. He still had his speech and could still tell stories about his days "pounding the pavement."

The nurses enjoyed Ben's tales of high living, particularly how he would wine and dine his clients at some of Boston's most famous seafood restaurants.

One day, in the retelling of one of those famous "deal-clinching luncheons," Ben got a hankering for lobster. "Boy, a boiled live lobster with butter sure would taste good!" he began to say to anybody who would listen. The more he talked about lobster, the more he wanted it.

Finally one of the staff went to the administrator of the home. "Ben wants a lobster for dinner," she said.

"Well, why don't you order him one?" the administrator suggested.

The night of the lobster dinner, Ben's eyes were shining like the sea itself. And judging from the eyes of the staff who were working that night, it was hard to say who enjoyed the evening the most. Everyone felt Ben's happiness.

Preparing for bed, Ben said, "I think I'll order lobster for the whole building!"

TODAY: Grant a wish.

The universal fears—we all know them: snakes, the dark, spiders, deep water. And as we get older another phobia joins the crowd—going to a nursing home.

For both the frail older person and her family, the thought of moving from home into a facility is often terrifying.

Rebecca E. Greer wrote in *Woman's Day* (July 1992) of her family's experience placing her eighty-nine-year-old mother into "a home." Of visiting her mother in the facility she says:

> Clearly she had not accepted the permanence of her situation. In truth, neither had I. My first hours in the home were agonizing. When Mom whispered, "Get me out of here," I briefly considered it. When she pleaded with me to overrule the "mean" aides who gently coaxed her to eat, I felt like a traitor for taking their side.
>
> As the months turned into years, my views of nursing homes changed. I became convinced my mother could not have lived as long or as comfortably anywhere else. She always dreaded becoming "a burden" to her children and found it easier to rely on hired help to meet her growing needs—especially when it meant cleaning a soiled bed after a bowel problem. Thanks to the sensitivity of her attendants, she kept her dignity. Even when she barely had the strength to lift a spoon, she still asked to be dressed and have makeup applied.

TODAY: Help take away fear.

Working in a nursing facility, it is easy to get caught up in a "bad news reporter" pattern. Staff spend time collecting evidence or information about what is bad at the facility and they devote plenty of energy to talking about it.

A variation of this theme is staff who like to talk about bad news at other facilities. "Did you hear what they make the aides do at Golden Manor?" is the opening question, and then the bad news flows.

Knowing that the general public has a real suspicion, even a fear, of nursing homes, it makes no sense to spread such stories. Gradually, as the bad news travels the stores and offices of a community, it changes, gets worse, gets mixed up. By spreading bad news, we do nothing to change the way others regard nursing homes or growing old.

Pretty soon the simple complaint that went out through the facility door is coming back through the window. Staff begin to hear about terrible things that are supposedly happening at their own workplace! "No, that's not what happened! And it didn't happen here anyway!" the staff cry, but it is too late. The damage has been done.

The best place to report bad news is to the person who can do something to improve the situation. Otherwise keep quiet.

TODAY: Bear no bad news.

Not being connected to others is one of our greatest fears. Even dogs feel insecure; watch a pet when his master leaves the room.

Maintaining real communication with the outside world is a challenge for residents of long term care facilities. After a while the walls of the building become the boundaries of a patient's world. The news is limited to those who live and work in the home, with little else getting through.

At Stratton House and Heins House, a nursing home and its sister residential care facility, the staff saw a way to connect with others that would bring meaning to the patients' lives.

Having mastered several dozen jigsaw puzzles, the residents didn't want to put the same puzzles together again. "New puzzles, please!" they cried. But the staff wondered what to do with the old, used-only-once, perfectly good puzzles. At last someone seized on the idea of donating the puzzles to the nearby correctional facility. "Those poor boys are more trapped than we are," a resident mused, proudly explaining how his puzzles were going to make others happy.

A formal presentation to one of the prison officials was arranged, with the photographer from the local newspaper there to publicize this moment of connection and generosity.

TODAY: Look for connections.

In America today it is trendy to talk about being comfortable with one's own death, to control even its time and place. Ever seeking full domination over the natural elements, we humans want to leave little to chance, to the Fates.

As in all businesses, entrepreneurs see opportunities to capitalize on the latest cultural trends, offering quick-fix workshops for virtually every marketable aspect of human life. Seminars and public talks on how to die and how to plan your own death are popping up everywhere.

Back in 1980, Rev. George Fitchette, chaplain supervisor at St. Luke's Medical Center in Chicago, wrote an article entitled "Wisdom and Folly in Death and Dying." Based on Psalm 90:12 ("So teach us to number our days that we may get a heart of wisdom"), the article speaks to the paradoxical nature of working with the dying. Rev. Fitchett suggests that, while Americans have become more comfortable with death, we have not become any wiser about it. "We must meditate on our own death in order to be wise," he writes. "We must reflect on our numbered days, our finitude." Not to do so, he argues, is to live in folly.

Taking his thinking one step further, Rev. Fichett believes it isn't possible for us to become comfortable with our own mortality. We hate the fact that life will end! It stinks! Rather, this chaplain maintains, "We have to become more comfortable with the discomfort that our own mortality and the experience of working with the dying will continually cause us."

Admit our fears? That is precisely what is suggested here. Only when we face and admit the impossibility of being comfortable with caring for the dying, will we be able to do just that.

TODAY: Accept impossibilities.

"I wish she had to do my job for just one day," the nurses' aide whispered. "Then we would have enough girls on this shift to take care of all these patients!"

How many of us have imagined our bosses trying to do our jobs? Particularly in our moments of frustration, we want them to feel the same exhaustion and hopelessness we do. We want them to see this trap we live in, and, maybe, to make things different.

Why not organize the staff and create an Administrator As Aide for the Afternoon (AAAA) day? Invite your administrator (and maybe other management, like the director of nursing) to spend four hours working as an aide some afternoon. Experience is the best teacher, and one such afternoon could be worth a thousand meetings.

When you extend your invitation, don't do it in bitterness or impatience. Be proud of your work and proud of what you bring to the lives of your patients. Welcome your administrator to experience the joys, as well as the sorrows, of your calling.

TODAY: Arrange an AAAA meeting.

What is healthcare reform? Most people think it means better service for less money.

As we've watched politicians and legislatures try to wrestle this monster, most Americans have realized the way to tackle a monster is one leg at a time. Outside of an earthquake or bankruptcy, step by step is the best recipe for real change.

At Union House Nursing Home in Glover, Vermont (a town of 800+ people), administrator Pat Russell read a lot about healthcare reform. What did it mean for her small facility and her small town?

Surveying her community and its healthcare needs, Pat quickly realized that there was one easy step toward reform that she could take without any governmental body's approval—she could offer office space to the visiting doctor. Once a week the physician visited the nursing home to examine its patients, while all other sick residents of Glover had to drive some twenty miles one way to the doctor's office in Newport. So Pat provided the doctor a room where he could see all his Glover patients—at the nursing home in Glover.

TODAY: Create reforms!

Famed anthropologist Dr. Ashley Montague has created a list of twenty-six traits essential to our growth and well-being. Is there any trait where you're down a pint? Any changes you deserve?

1. Ability to love.
2. The need for friendship.
3. Sensitivity.
4. The ability to think soundly.
5. The need to learn.
6. The need to work.
7. The need to know.
8. The need to organize.
9. Curiosity.
10. A sense of wonder.
11. Playfulness.
12. Imagination.
13. Creativity.
14. Open-mindedness.
15. Flexibility.
16. The willingness to experiment.
17. Explorativeness.
18. Resilience.
19. Optimism.
20. Joyfulness.
21. The ability to express emotions.
22. Honesty and trust.
23. Sense of humor.
24. Compassion.
25. The ability to enjoy dancing.
26. The ability to enjoy singing.

TODAY: Where do you deserve to grow?

Dust to dust. You can't take it with you. Money can't buy you love.

We all pay lip service to the notion that consuming things, that shopping till we drop, is not the secret to our happiness. But we also will run into burning buildings to rescue a family picture or a piece of heirloom jewelry.

Our affection for things is not so much for the material as for the sentimental. We love what the thing represents, what it symbolizes.

At the Converse Home in Burlington—a lovely old mansion that is now home to some twenty retired women—a custom is practiced that honors the memories of residents who die. Recognizing the value of symbols, the home plants a tree or a shrub in the name of each resident who has passed away. This Memory Garden is a living memorial to lives well lived and to the contributions of Vermont women.

For visiting family and friends, a stroll through the special landscape triggers all kinds of conversation and emotions. Through this simple gesture, the Converse Home provides those who grieve and love with a focus, a tangible place to cherish their memories.

TODAY: See symbols.

Thankfully, the state of the art in health care for dementia patients is, as much as possible, to let them be free. Suffering from a terminal brain disorder and being confined to a healthcare facility are enough of an adjustment—without the added injury of being tied to a chair.

Yet all staff recognize that the patient labeled "wanderer" can make life stressful and difficult in a nursing home. Chasing patients, untangling them from each other, returning missing personal property and bandaging bruises become standard staff responsibilities. Perhaps inconvenient for staff and other residents, it's still a fair trade for those who would otherwise be tied up.

Despite all of the security systems and staff in-services on dealing with wanderers, some manage to get out of the building. (In official in-service programs, these patients take on a new label: elopers!) When it already seems there aren't enough staff to provide care inside the building, how will staff be spared to go on a treasure hunt?

Innovative nurses like Anne Johnson create a Frequent Flyer Program with their facility's neighbors. Pictures of the wandering residents are distributed to the houses and offices nearby, and neighbors are taught how to graciously return a confused resident to the nursing home. Residents prone to walking also wear little name tags that ask strangers to help them find their way back.

TODAY: Know your neighbors!

Milton was so agitated. "Terrible, terrible, terrible!" he would bellow, gazing off into an unknown time and space. A retired telephone company employee, Milton was suffering from some form of dementia. Confined to a wheelchair, wearing a diaper, Milton didn't know he was living in a nursing home.

In Milton's mind, he was stuck on vacation away from home, trying to get back to Pennsylvania, a good one thousand mile drive from where he was. Like an endless loop tape, Milton would begin with his "terrible" chant, adding, "This is no good; I've got to go."

One day I visited to make bead angels with the staff and patients. Hearing Milton's constant bellowing, I asked the staff what was wrong. "He is always like that; we can't do anything for him," I was told. Unlike the staff, I hadn't become oblivious to Milton's wails: "I can't stand that noise! Bring him here!"

Once at the table, I began to ask Milton what was so terrible. He explained he had been away from home for almost four weeks and it was time to get back. For the next hour, we talked about Milton's work, travels and family. I repeatedly asked Milton questions, praised him for his accomplishments, reassured him he could go home "as soon as the roads clear up." Several times Milton broke into tears.

After dinner, with Milton's distress still on my mind, I dropped by the old man's room. "Milton, I would like to pray with you tonight. Let's pray that you don't feel upset anymore, that you find some peace." He looked shocked when I said the words "upset" and "peace." Holding hands, we sat and prayed.

Six hours later, for no apparent reason, Milton died in his sleep. Looking back on the day, the social services director said, "I have never heard Milton talk so much. I think it was very healing for him." Milton was able spiritually to settle.

TODAY: Listen to heal.

My grandmother's nursing home, Braintree Manor in Braintree, Massachusetts, has just converted a visiting parlor into a pub, complete with bar. Two or three nights a week, my Gram can go and have lovely appetizers and some wine. Hearing her describe the event, I know it's a hit.

In his book *Alcohol and Old Age* (1980), C. M. Steele reports of a study of the effectiveness of alcohol as a social lubricant on residents of a nursing home. It seems that, two months after the hospital staff began offering an afternoon beer to the geriatric patients, the number of them who could walk on their own increased from 21 percent to 74 percent. Social interaction tripled, and the percentages of patients taking Thorazine, a strong tranquilizer, dropped from 75 percent to zero!

Never underestimate the power of a glass of sherry.

TODAY: Open a pub!

In celebration of Thanksgiving Day, here is a poem written by Ed Welch, a resident at the Vermont Veterans Home in Bennington.

Thank You For This Day

Good morning Lord, it's only me
I've come to have a talk with thee.
First of all, I'd like to say
Thank you Lord, for this beautiful day.
For home, food and loving care
For all the goodness everywhere.
It's nice to know you're always there
Each time I come to you in prayer.
Thank you for the flowers
That bloom in early spring
Thank you for the little birds
And the songs they bring.

And for the lovely rose bush
That grows right by my door,
Thank you Lord for all these things
And a million more.
I'd like you to know how I feel
And that my love for you is real.
I've got so much I'd like to say
As I talk to you my God today.
Oh, it's such a pretty day today;
The sun shines down on me.
It's such a pretty day today
For all the world to see.
What would I do without you
I need you more each day,
To help me get back on my feet
When I fall along the way.
I've done so much to be thankful for,
I don't know where to start.
All I can say is thank you Lord
From the bottom of my heart.

TODAY: Find a poet.

Every family, every office, every nursing home has its own customs, traditions, standards and practices. Some folks work as a team, pitching in when they are needed. Others have well organized charts, showing who does what and when. There is no one good way for all situations, but rather good ways for each situation.

What is the standard and practice in your nursing home for answering a call button? How much time do you let pass before you answer the light or bell? How much time is too much time to wait?

Director of Nursing Anne Johnson, whom you met on November 22, played a little game with her staff to emphasize the importance of answering the patient's call button.

Sitting on the toilet of a resident's room, Anne pulled the cord for help. And waited. And waited. And waited. An aide finally showed up, snapping "What do you want?" As she opened the door, Anne answered, "You."

Knowing their boss might be waiting in the toilet, the staff began to move more quickly when patients rang for help. After a while the facility shifted its standard from a several minute wait to a very short wait.

TODAY: Answer patient calls.

Looking forward to the first day of school in the fall, or a new job, can cause butterflies. But these beginnings cannot compare to the mixed emotions that churn on the day one moves into the nursing home. Since we all think we are going to avoid such a stay, it comes as quite a shock. About one of every five people will spend time in a nursing home during their lifetime. But nobody thinks they will be that one; we all fully expect to be one of the other four!

At Woodridge, the nursing home associated with Central Vermont Hospital in Berlin, the staff was dissatisfied with how they handled admissions. They evaluated their process and found it was heavy on paperwork and very light on hospitality. Committed to improving this traumatic day's impact on new patients, the staff launched a lengthy review and design project. The goal? To create a new, friendlier, more comfortable first day at Woodridge.

Other facilities have conducted similar self-analyses and discovered some obvious but still startling practices. Imagine! Some homes found that they were routinely giving baths to patients on their first day. Already reeling from the changes and losses, why should any patient have to deal with becoming naked before a stranger? Homes that had this practice decided waiting to bathe patients for a day or two wouldn't rock the world.

TODAY: Review Day One.

The Bible tells us we cannot be prophets in our own land. People cannot hear wisdom from us whom they see every day, for we lack the shimmer of the consultant. To find guidance and advice for daily living, they go to be lectured by famous people, believing they'll have the needed answers.

In their book *The Feminine Face of God,* Sherry Ruth Anderson and Patricia Hopkins tell us this:

> To find our connection to the ancient grandmothers or to elders from another time or culture is sometimes easier than to appreciate the gifts we have received from our own immediate family: our mothers and aunts and grandmothers.

The two describe a lecture given by Seneca Indian Yehwehnode, an elder in the Wolf Clan. After her talk, a young woman approached Yehwehnode: "It is such a gift to hear your wisdom, Grandmother. How I wish we had others like you! But we have no crones, no elders."

The Indian leader replied, "Yes you do. You've stuffed them out of sight in old age homes. You can't hear what they have to say. You can't receive what is already in front of you...Start now to acknowledge those who help you and love you. Show your gratitude."

TODAY: Show your gratitude.

The average patient in a nursing home is eighty-five years of age. She has seen great changes in her lifetime—from automobiles, to telephones, to televisions, to computers. Beyond the technological advances, the world has become a place with more deadly weapons, broken families and shifts in the roles of men and women.

While all of us feel somewhat powerless in the face of the evening news, the daunting nature of the changing society can be overwhelming for those who are frail and dependent. We all wonder how we can make a difference, how we can take away some of the planet's pain. No longer working, or even paying taxes, the nursing home patient can quickly feel like just another example of the culture's collapse, more of a burden than anything else.

One such way to beat this sense of uselessness is through volunteering with the At risk Baby Crib quilt project (ABC). This national volunteer effort sends homemade blankets to the thousands of small children around the world who are infected with the HIV/AIDS virus, are HIV+, or born addicted.

Volunteers are asked to make quilts 36" x 36"—just right for a crib. Most communities have churches that coordinate the ABC project. In Vermont, call Susan Stewart (802-893-8261). Nursing homes are full of former quilters. Perhaps they could create a quilt that will swaddle a needy baby?

TODAY: Help a resident volunteer.

Consider the words of Nadine Stair:

If I had to live my life over, I'd like to make more mistakes next time. I'd relax. I would limber up. I would be sillier than I have been this trip. I would take fewer things seriously. I would take more chances. I would climb more mountains and swim more rivers...I would have more actual troubles, but I'd have fewer imaginary ones.

You see, I'm one of those people who live sensibly and sanely hour after hour, day after day. Oh, I've had my moments. And if I had to do it over again, I'd have more of them. In fact, I'd try to have nothing else. Just moments, one after another, instead of living so many years ahead of each day. I've been one of those persons who never goes anywhere without a ther-mometer, a hot water bottle, a raincoat, and a parachute. If I had to do it again, I would travel lighter than I have.

If I had my life to live over, I would start barefoot earlier in the spring and stay that way later in the fall. I would go to more dances. I would ride more merry-go-rounds. I would pick more daisies.

TODAY: Don't wait to do it over again.

December

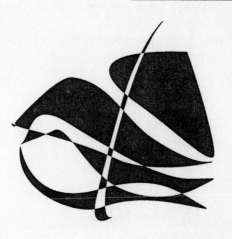

December 1

The ways we say "I'm here" range from singing to writing poetry to hunting to gardening and beyond. When she was nine years old, Priscilla Hood of Duxbury discovered poetry was a way she could express herself and make sense of her world.

A lifetime later, as a patient at Rowan Court Nursing Home, Priscilla wrote this:

It was April 17, 1990
That I changed my wearing apparel
To one of these nighties.
Has no buttons on
But in the back—strings.
When you could not sleep
You thought of lots of things
You couldn't get into bed alone,
And you cried because
You had to sell your home.
I, like everyone here,
cry inside, but laugh—
seems so queer.
What would I do
If I wasn't in a place like this?
I wouldn't have any care,
or with others their troubles share.
Here, always, will be my home,
So I will never be alone.

TODAY: Listen for crying behind the laughter.

We are now at the beginning of Advent season, the time of year Christians prepare for the birth of the Baby Jesus. For the Jews, this is the time of Hanukkah. And for the secular world, it is a time of buying gifts and planning parties. For all of us, December is a month of good tidings.

You, as a caregiver, are among those who carry the message of caring year round, not just during these winter holidays. Working in the US, you are living among people who are more prone to violence that any other industrialized nation.

In 1980 there were eight handgun murders in England, compared to 10,012 in the US.

Your work is a powerful force for good and peace in the world. Continue to touch with tenderness, to forgive with frequency, to laugh with joy. In a time and place where hurting one another is ho-hum news, you are the bright star in the east.

TODAY: Be a peacemaker.

December 3

Growing old is not something to do alone. But for many people living in your facility, that is what they are doing.

Having spent twenty, thirty, or even fifty years of their lives in mental health institutions, they long ago lost their connections to town. Families kept their distance, and friendships were never made.

What do they have to look forward to? Simple things.

Like learning to sleep in a bed instead of strapped into a reclining chair. Or better still, sleeping with the door shut and lights out. Big mental hospitals often were lit all night long, and doors had to be open.

For others it may be enjoying a more interesting menu, actually putting on some weight and feeling stronger. With interesting food and loving hands to feed them, people can gain weight and strength.

Old age is more than falling or choking, the two leading causes of death for those over ninety. Old age is life, and, with your help, it can be well lived.

TODAY: Share aging.

Many caregivers have discovered the special messages of the dying—special because they are often delivered in a certain way, almost coded. In your day-to-day interactions with patients, such messages may arrive without notice or fanfare. That's why you need to know the language, to be able to translate the message.

In their published work, registered nurses Patricia Kelley and Maggie Callanan refer to themes being communicated by dying patients. The five categories which they find people most frequently speaking from are:

❖ being in the presence of, or talking to, someone who is not alive
❖ preparing for travel or change
❖ describing a place other than the one they are in
❖ needing reconciliation
❖ knowing when death will occur

For example, if a dying patient begins to tell you they need a map to get home, instead of dismissing their words as hallucinations or confusion, listen for the special message. Assure the patient she will find her way home, that it is okay to go. Watch their anxiety and frustration disappear.

TODAY: Understand special messages.

Nursing homes are not Hollywood productions. If only there were producers and directors with scriptwriters who made sure every day had a happy ending!

When your patients are mainly those with a dementia, longing for Hollywood is especially easy. Trying to explain something to someone who is no longer able to understand the basics of time, date and place is a thankless, often hopeless, exercise.

For staff in one small facility, a character of this type was Mr. Grimby. A former landlord, Mr. Grimby was often roaming the nursing home halls barking at the other residents, "You're out of here! I'm evicting you! Now!" The ensuing confusion defied description. Everyone got upset following an eviction!

While it was funny on one level, staff couldn't let it go. Gently taking Mr. Grimby aside, they would speak to him clearly about the patients around him being there because of health problems. They would then remind him that he too had some health problems. While this explanation calmed him a bit, he still needed a diversion. A cookie usually worked well, though he gained ten pounds in three months with this script!

TODAY: Create some happy endings.

One of the largest women's groups in the world is the Business and Professional Women's Club. When gathered, the women recite what they call a collect, like a short prayer, written by Mary Stewart. It reads:

Keep us, O God, from pettiness; let us be large in thought, in word, in deed. Let us be done with fault-finding and leave off self-seeking.

May we put away all pretense and meet each other face to face—without self-pity and without prejudices. May we never be hasty in judgment and always generous.

Let us take time for all things; make us grow calm, serene and gentle. Teach us to put into action our better impulses, straightforward and unafraid.

Grant that we may realize it is the little things that create difference, that in the big things of life we are at one.

And may we strive to touch and to know the great, common human heart of us all; and, O Lord God, let us forget not to be kind!

TODAY: Write a facility collect with others.

Never underestimate the power of one nursing home employee who decides something needs to be done.

Outside of Cleveland, Ohio, is the town of Milan. There, at the Edison healthcare Center, activities director Carolyn Walton works hard at making the days meaningful for her patients. That's why she kept wondering why Mary Volanti never had any visitors. Mary's records indicated she had a son, so Carolyn asked her about her son.

"His name is Charles," said Mary, who also told Carolyn the date of Charles's birthday.

With the help of a coworker who does genealogy research, Carolyn Walton got a computer program with national phone listings. She called the three Charles Volantis, but none was Mary's son. One, though, was Charles's cousin, and he told her Charles lived in Olympia, Washington.

When Carolyn called Olympia and was told the number was unpublished, she persevered, convincing an operator to leave a message for Charles about his mother.

A few hours later, Charles, aged fifty-four, called. At age six he had been told by his father that his mom had died. "I have a mommy?" he asked, stunned.

Thanks to a persistent nursing home employee, mother and son have been reunited and have pledged never to lose touch again.

TODAY: Wonder about visitors.

A peek inside the mailbag of The Arbors, a special dementia facility in Shelburne:

> God bless you for creating the Arbors. It was a loving home for Mother's final years, providing her with the finest quality care and providing me with the opportunity to share the most loving, positive experiences of my life. You are to be commended for the superb staff you have brought together; they are truly love in action. During my extended stay I witnessed the compassion, gentle humor and dignity each resident received. I sensed a commitment much deeper than doing a "job." Mother and I gained a very special second family.

and

> Thank you, each and everyone, for the devoted, loving care you bestowed on Mother. You walked the final mile with her and gently ushered her into Heaven. Even in the depths of her illness you caught the magic of her true personality.

and

> Last Wednesday and Thursday were possibly the most difficult twenty-four hours of my life and each of you surrounded me with emotional pillows. Words cannot begin to describe how much each of you helped.

TODAY: Be an emotional pillow.

Time for a reality check. This is a nursing home, with equal emphasis on its first and last name. Sometimes, when the most important focus of the day becomes checking off your list of duties, the last name, home, shrinks in importance.

Like the day the staff sent the cable TV man into Mrs. Bunting's room. Seems hers was the last room to connect to the cable system, and Mr. Cable wanted to get the work done so he could finally leave the building.

No one thought about the fact that Mrs. Bunting was perched on the bed pan. Or that the curtains weren't drawn. Or that her privacy was being completely violated by a stranger.

And the poor cable man. He felt weird, but thought the staff must know better. Around Mrs. Bunting's room and floor he crawled.

How would you like to have been Mrs. Bunting?

TODAY: Remember your facility's last name.

Most of the miraculous workings of the human body remain a mystery. Just how the brain functions is unclear, as are the the workings of the complex, marvelous immune system.

What we do know about immunity is that when people are grieving, or alone, or sad, their immune system declines. When they feel connected to the community, the immune system improves, thus assuring a better chance of survival for the individual and the society at large.

What happens to the immune systems of caregivers? After all, you are often exposed to contagious diseases and other threats to your health.

A study at Harvard University showed that just the watching of caregivers can improve the immune system. Students viewed a film on the life of one of the greatest caregivers of all time, Mother Teresa (see January 30). In stark footage, Mother Teresa was shown caring for the sick and dying of Calcutta.

In tests conducted after the movie, the students were found to have enhanced immunity. Even students who said they felt no sympathy for the work of Mother Teresa had improved immune system functioning.

Perhaps it is time for you to talk about your caregiving with friends. Who knows? Listening to you might improve their health!

TODAY: Improve everyone's immunity.

A retired physician who worked in northern Vermont and in mental health clinics in New Hampshire, Dr. Emily T. Wilson, has some strong opinions about the use of restraints in nursing homes. Living at one of the famed Kendal continuing care retirement communities, she agreed to appear on a Kendal videotape speaking about patient autonomy, and particularly the use of physical restraints. Dr. Wilson said:

> The use of physical restraints is in direct opposition to the principle of autonomy. It is imposed upon confused, inarticulate, difficult people who are given no choice in the matter. But I think the whole problem goes beyond the concept of autonomy: Restraint is an insult to, an attack upon, the unique spirit of a human being; it treats him as less than human; it manipulates him; it destroys his self-respect.

Continuing her talk, Dr. Wilson explored the question of what goes on in the human mind when the patient is apparently comatose or otherwise unable or unwilling to communicate:

> The more I have observed such people, the more certain I am that something is going on, and we dare not forget that as we consider their treatment…. They may be restless and difficult to handle, but they most certainly do not need the burden of adjusting to physical restraint during this period of critical spiritual searching. No one really knows, but because no one knows, no one should dare to interfere.

TODAY: Try not to interfere in anyone's spiritual search.

Do you wonder about wanderers?

Such patients can test your patience, but, if you take a minute, their seemingly aimless shuffling and pacing can begin to make sense. By becoming a careful observer of wanderers, you can make life for everyone a lot more comfortable.

Other caregivers who have watched wanderers have drawn certain conclusions:

❖ People wander for many reasons.
❖ The first and last rooms on a corridor hold a certain appeal.
❖ Sometimes their body knows they are looking for a bathroom, but they can't express this need.
❖ Other times, hunger can get them out of their chairs and into the halls, but, again, they can't tell you.

Still others may be triggered to walk because they see someone put on a coat or boots or gloves. For those who suffer under severe short term memory loss, their minds return to memories that are clear, to times when they had responsibilities: "I have to meet the school bus." "I've got to bring my husband his lunch pail." The patients will feel the need to do something that was a common occurrence in their younger years, as it is familiar and comfortable.

Caregivers who try to convince such wanderers that their children are grown up and living in another state will usually just make the patients more upset and agitated. It is better to tell your wanderers that the kids are getting off the bus at a friend's today, and that the lunch pail was already delivered. Always seek to bring peace and comfort.

TODAY: Wonder about wanderers.

Ever meet anyone with zeal? Real zeal? Like the stars of those infomercials on television? How could one mop make so many women so excited?! Zeal in a nursing home can show up when it is least desired. Reading the actual language of the law that calls for nursing homes to help patients "attain and maintain their highest level of functioning," some nurses can push pretty hard.

Alice was 104 years old. She had lived to this ripe old age as a wife and mother who even taught piano lessons and Sunday School in her day. Now, after living 103 years independently in the community, she needed a nursing home. Moving into the healthcare facility, Alice wasn't afraid or bitter or depressed or angry. She was just tired out.

The zealous care plan called for Alice to gain the ability to walk fifty feet each day and then to maintain it. After all, didn't the federal government demand it? It made sense to the staff, and even to Alice's eighty-year-old daughter. But not to Alice.

"I'm 104 years old. I've done all the walking I want. I came here to rest, and that's what I'm going to do," she told the staff. She spent the remainder of her days in bed or in a wheelchair, quite content.

TODAY: What do your patients want?

Memorial services are becoming more and more common place in nursing homes. Whether formal or informal, involving outsiders or just the staff, residents and volunteers, such services can help everyone deal with death and move on.

Poems, memories and stories can be read, and a few hymns sung. Sometimes candles are lit in memory of those loved ones who have died. Sometimes funny recollections are shared, allowing laughter to heal the broken hearts. A favorite verse to read at such services is called "Miss Me, But Let Me Go."

When I come to the end of the road
And the sun has set for me
I want no rites in a gloom filled room;
Why cry for a soul set free?
Miss me a little, but not too long,
And not with your head bowed low.
Remember the love that we once shared;
Miss me, but let me go.
For this is a journey that we all must take
And each must go alone.
It's all part of the Master's plan,
A step on the road to home.
When you are lonely and sick of heart
Go to the friends we know
And bury your sorrows in doing good deeds;
Miss me, but let me go.

TODAY: Toast some memories.

Marilyn had a long and wickedly hard day as an aide. Coworkers had called in sick and she had to cover their assignments. She felt a cold coming on and by dinner time found herself flat on her back on her living room couch.

A single mom with three sons, Marilyn didn't have much help at home either.

"Mom, can we decorate the Christmas tree tonight?" asked her youngest, excited about the season. The family had bought their tree earlier, and it was sitting on the front porch.

Exhausted, Marilyn groaned and said, "Well, OK. You bring the tree in and I'll get the decorations from the attic."

"Can't you bring the tree in too?" the kids whined, staring at the television.

Marilyn blew. "I'm canceling Christmas," she yelled. "I'm sick of doing everything myself. Grabbing a hatchet, she went out onto the porch and chopped the tree into pieces.

Looking back on the day, Marilyn saw that she had let resentment build up. She had allowed herself to feel taken advantage of and victimized at work; consequently, her family had suffered, and so had Marilyn. A healthier response to her stress would have been to tell her kids that she needed some extra help, that she was hurting.

TODAY: Express your needs honestly.

GUARDIAN ANGELS
By the Patient Poetry Circle, Gill Home, Ludlow

You are the ones
who treat us as older sisters
who tell us what's going on
in your homes.
You are the ones
whose hands massage us
when we dress and always
it feels so good on our legs.
You are the ones
who help us—
after a whirlpool bath and lotion
we feel a whole year younger.
You are the ones
who compliment our hair and clothes,
who take pains
to talk gently to us
even when we complain.
Late at night
we'll see your shadow
on the curtains.
Three times a night
with your little flashlight
you check to see if we're restless:
Are you all right?
Do you need help—or Tylenol?
You call us by our own first names.
You know our ways, always
our Guardian Angels.

TODAY: Be a Guardian Angel.

It seems talking about sex is not easy whatever our age.

As teenagers, we wanted information, but couldn't bear to ask our parents. Our parents wanted to give us information, but they felt just about as awkward as we did approaching the topic.

In a nursing facility, as in any place where people are gathered, sex and sexuality need to be talked about; yet everybody still feels pretty uncomfortable.

An attractive, thirty-three-year-old activities director once sighed, "My eighty-year-old residents want me to counsel them about sex. I haven't even gotten my own sex life figured out!"

Remember: Happily, romance can occur in a nursing home. Uphold the patients' right to make choices and be given privacy. Remember to approach each situation with respect, striving to preserve their dignity.

Among the dementia population, the sex drive seems to have declined. Sometimes masturbation occurs in public. Placing pillows over a patient's lap may prevent the activity. Dressing a woman in pants instead of a skirt is also wise, and can help her avoid the tendency to expose herself.

TODAY: Respect your patient's sexual nature.

What are the words we associate with aging? Arthritis, heart attack, stroke, dementia, falling. Not a pretty picture.

Rabbi Zalman Schachter-Shalomi, the director of the Spiritual Eldering Project based in Philadelphia, chooses very different words when speaking of aging.

He leads workshops on sageing, which the Rabbi defines as coming to grips with this important time in our lives, affirming the success of a long life, opening up to questions about the meaning of life and reconciling lifelong struggles. The goal of Spiritual Eldering is to free the elder to live in the present by expanding awareness and increasing appetite for life.

Ultimately, when American society comes to see aging as the wonderful gift that it is, we will think of the wisdom and the life experiences associated with becoming old, not the physical infirmities. And when that day comes, we will see you, the caregivers of the aged, as precious people whose work is a privilege.

TODAY: Promote sageing.

Have you heard the hiss in the lounge?
It
topples governments,
wrecks marriages,
ruins careers,
busts reputations,
causes heartaches,
nightmares,
indigestion,
spawns suspicion,
generates grief,
dispatches innocent people
to cry
in their pillows.
Even its name
hisses.
It's called
gossip.

Office gossip,
Shop gossip.
Party gossip.
It makes
headlines
and headaches.
Before
you repeat
a story,
ask yourself:
Is it true?
Is it fair?
Is it necessary?
If not,
shut up.

TODAY: Stop gossip.

December 20

Is there a classroom, church choir or Girl Scout troop that hasn't made the rounds of your facility this holiday season?

Seems every group magically discovers nursing homes this month. Though there is a shortage of visitors the other eleven months of the year, December brings company. Families, friends and well-meaning civic groups arrive with gifts, candy and song. Some days it can almost be too much.

Nationally, The Holiday Project coordinates visits to all kinds of institutions, including nursing homes, on Christmas Day itself. This unusual gesture can make a wonderful impression on patients. Few other folks like to leave the comfort of their homes on Christmas Day. And, if you happen to be working this Christmas, remind your visitors that the other 364 days of the year are just as lonely for your patients. If you have time, explain how non-holidays are even quieter, that visits would be particularly appreciated on Any Old Day.

TODAY: Welcome visitors.

Today (or near this date) is the Winter Solstice, a day celebrated for centuries by people around the world. Today marks the beginning of winter; from now on the days begin to grow shorter.

For those whose lives are lived more indoors than outdoors, the shortened days of sun can have a negative effect. No longer does a window provide lots of sun and cheerfulness. Gray skies become the standard, and the mornings are dark.

The heliotrope is a beautiful flower that has a unique pattern. It actually moves to follow the sun. If the sun is in the east, the flower turns its bloom to face due east. When the sun heads west, the flower does too.

These cold, dark days, think of your patients as heliotropes. They may not know how to follow the sun, but they would like to feel its warmth. Your job can be to wheel their chairs to a different, sunny spot in the building, where they can enjoy the precious daylight. Like little heliotropes, they will bloom and shine in the light.

TODAY: Help your heliotropes.

"I'm a recreational therapist specializing in social and interactive modalities."

Huh? The translation? "I talk to patients to help them feel happy."

Sometimes the over-professionalizing of a job can make it downright silly and top-heavy. Caregivers can get caught up in their titles, be they certified, licensed or registered, and forget the basics.

Paperwork becomes the goal, rather than listening to a patient, or telling a cute story, or braiding someone's hair.

Bosses who make their roles and training seem so important and intimidating can make you forget your worth. Don't forget what the patient wants and needs, because she is the true boss. Education and workshops and knowledge are necessary, but not as necessary as a caring, compassionate heart. Without love, no amount of book learning makes a difference.

As the Buddhist monk Thich Nhat Hanh wrote: "Waking up this morning, I smile. Twenty-four brand new hours before me. I vow to live fully each moment and to look at all beings with eyes of compassion."

TODAY: Look through eyes of compassion.

Feeling like you can't possibly get it all done? Work, shop, wrap gifts, fill the stockings, cook the turkey, decorate the tree? It is an unbelievable assignment and one that only a woman would think reasonable!

In your next life, why not consider returning as a bird, specifically, as a Wilson's Phalarope? She has truly got it made.

Unlike most of the rest of the bird kingdom, where males are the most beautifully colored and feathered, the female Wilson's is more gorgeous than her mate. But her advantage doesn't stop there. She courts her husband openly, with high-flying aerial antics and musical water ballets in which she swims toward the males with her neck feathers all ruffled singing a chugging song. At times several females will chase one male.

But her outrageousness gets better. After mating, he sits on the eggs and she takes off! And when the babies hatch, he feeds them, while she sometimes leaves, or sometimes stays, carefree, splashing in the shallow waters.

So when someone asks what you wish for Christmas, tell them you wish you were a Wilson's Phalarope.

TODAY: Be a little phalaropeish.

December 24

We know one of the ways that people stay mentally well is through their connections with others. Family and friends remind us of who we are, what we are. Another truth involves seeing how much better off you are than someone else. Seeing someone who has no legs humbles the person complaining about aching feet.

Perhaps governed by these truths, or maybe even by a greater sense of compassion, the administrator of a small Connecticut nursing home, Lorraine Franco, embarked upon a Christmas service project some years ago that exposed her patients to a changing world of pain and suffering.

Lorraine decided to help her patients help the prisoners in a nearby state correctional facility. The nursing home patients crocheted Christmas stockings and filled them with goodies. Some of the goodies were condoms. Why condoms?

"Because as a healthcare worker I know the dangers of transmitting diseases, particularly AIDS," said the straightforward Lorraine. She said the project and conversations that it generated among her patients were tremendous. Patients felt meaningfully connected to the suffering of others, as well as the vulnerabilities of being human.

TODAY: Reach beyond your walls.

A wonderfully creative LPN named Mary Anne Pitman of the Flora Care Center wrote a variation on "'Twas The Night Before Christmas." It tells of Santa's visit to the nursing home:

> "This is my last stop, I saved the best for last.
> I brought every resident a dream from the past.
> Tonight as they sleep, their smiles you will see.
> Each will be remembering their Christmases
>   previously."
> Santa continues, talking to the staff,
> "You're all very special, you're appreciated too;
> Where would their lives be if it wasn't for you?
> To each and every member of your staff
> I give you the gift of being able to laugh.
> The joy you bring to each resident each day
> Is worth more than money, more than I
>   can say.
> And now I must leave, I must go back and rest.
> But before I leave I have one last request.
> Hope, joy and love in each stocking I placed
> Please remove some each day and add to
>   your pace.
> The feelings you share could be all that
>   they see;
> Do it for them, for you and for me."

TODAY: Have a Merry Christmas!

Dealing with repetition is one of life's most annoying lessons.

Think of children who keep asking for something, or patients who chant the same question hour after hour. Those caregivers who spend most of their time with the demented have to learn lots of tricks and magic to deal with the normal frustration such repetition causes.

Melva Wickman, of Santa Barbara, California, has written (*Guideposts,* September, 1993) about the frustration and exhaustion she felt dealing with her husband Al's suffering due to Alzheimer's.

"How could I possibly deal with this!" she cried, alone one night.

Melva testifies that in her prayers, and for the next few weeks whenever she asked God for help, she would get answers. When Al would keep asking her what she was doing, she just hugged him instead of answering him. When he would pester her, she would kiss him, recalling her first wonderful date with him. And when she felt incredibly sad, watching her husband's mind disappear before her, she learned to laugh with him. Each time she used love and laughter, her husband would relax and smile.

The day came when Al moved to a nursing home. Melva came by every day to help with his care. One day she heard Al shouting; she found him fighting two male aides who were trying to get him to sit down.

I came close to Al and put my lips next to his ear. "I love you," I murmured. Al immediately quieted down and gently pressed his head against my mouth. Then he calmly sat in the chair, looked up at me and beamed.

TODAY: When repetition or frustration arise, try love.

P.S. Remember, poinsettias are poisonous when eaten. Watch your confused patients; the red leaves look good.

You don't have to have all the answers.

Isn't that great news? You don't have to have all the answers.

In fact, in the work you're in, you've got to see that you're here to learn. Everyday, every patient, every situation is different. There are few formulas to follow, few ready-made recipes for success. In her book *A Gentle Death,* Elizabeth Callari, RN, writes of what she does as a counselor and caregiver of the dying, but everything she says applies to those who work with the living, too.

She writes of successful caregivers, not giving a recipe, but a description:

> The most successful caregivers have been good, ordinary people who understand the profound truth that neither they nor anyone else can plant corn and then harvest tomatoes. That is, fury doesn't bring calm, nor resentment, cooperation; fear cannot command knowledge and contempt does not lead to love. To work with the dying (or living) is to step in an emotional field where these dichotomies and others must be felt, for they often defy logic. Advanced levels of education and training emphasize analysis and logic, which is the last thing dying (living) people need. Instead, those facing death (life) need the love and respect which affirm human worth and dignity.

TODAY: You don't have to know all the answers.

Two cute ideas to jazz up your day.

At Holiday House in St. Albans, each staff person is assigned a resident to visit with for twenty minutes daily for six weeks. That means everyone, including the non-care staff such as laundry, kitchen and maintenance.

The visiting can take place when it is convenient, but it is every day. The subject of the visiting is anything the pair wants to talk about. Great friendships have been born through this simple plan. And when the six weeks are up, the staff often refuse to switch to another patient. They don't want to stop visiting with their new friend.

Over at Woodridge in Berlin, at the 3 p.m. shift change, all staff must participate in small play groups. Having found that this late afternoon time of confusion is when many falls and accidents occur, the facility decided to create some programming for fifteen minutes. Even the administrator must play, be it tossing a ball or giving manicures.

Not surprisingly, the office staff and others who never get a chance to mingle with patients are especially keen on the play period. And the residents enjoy the new faces and extra attention.

TODAY: Make a new friend.

Some insight from Elizabeth C. Beyor, a resident of The Manor, Morrisville:

In childhood, we dreamed of wide-open futures, of limitless opportunities.

Emerging from a sheltered youth, we brought our lives into focus, pursued reality, lifted our sights and shaped our ideals.

During the middle years of adulthood, we tested our ideals against our expanding knowledge and experience. Our outlook widened and our vision shifted from the personal to the universal.

Suddenly, mayhap without warning, we find that we have grown old, and once again, as in our early years, the future is wide-open and glorious beyond all physical powers of perception. We stand before a door that opens into cosmic reality. Beyond that door there is peace.

Shortly, all of us will be pushed though that door, and the pain and sorrow and the limitations of mortality will be lifted from our souls. We will know then with surety that we have passed from death unto life.

This physical world is the dream, the detour mankind has had to take on the way to becoming like the gods. The future, bursting with life and love and achievement, is expanding to make room for the human race.

May the peace of God be within you all the way.

TODAY: See the wide-open future.

Believe in yourself.
Believe in your instincts about caring and loving.
Believe in your part of creation, to be creative today.
Celebrate your life.
Celebrate this day.
Celebrate the goodness around you.

TODAY: Believe in yourself. Celebrate your life.

New Year's Eve. A time of reflection and resolution, looking backward and forward.

Your patients have seen many more midnights on Times Square than you have. They have more to reflect upon, perhaps less to resolve.

At mealtime toast one another, what you've been through, what is to come. At Berlin Health and Rehabilitation Center, the New Year's Party is this afternoon, complete with a live band and champagne. The appetizers are served by staff in party dresses, and confetti abounds. Activities staffer Pam Prue takes her teeth out and dresses up in a diaper, playing the part of the New Year Baby.

The only thing that is different from any other New Year's party is that the clock strikes midnight at 3 p.m. That works best for the schedule and everyone is awake to enjoy the party. After all, the clock really means little on this night, so why not make it work for everyone?

TODAY: Happy New Year!

P.S. Send me your stories, poems, and inspiration for Volume II. My address is:

> Bethany Knight, LNA
> RR 2 Box 36
> Glover, VT 05839

Credits

Thanks to David Bryan and Annie Scarff, for their assistance with editing. Author's photo by Bethany Dunbar. Cover art is an original oil painting by Karen Cole. Patience and cheering by Thurmond Knight. Reality checks by Elliot Kaiman. Inspiration by Rhonda, Denise, Donna, Toni, Janet, Bridget, Deb, Sherrie, Arthur, Helen, Jeane, Ludie Mae, Carolyn, Tanya, Dawn, Wendie, David, Julia, Miss Jo Ann, Lynne, Melissa, Cathy, Linda, Lisa, James, Heather and all of the other holy members of this nation's royal family of spiritual healers.

Thank You

The publisher would like to thank the Beverly Foundation and its President Helen Kerschner for their generous encouragement and financial support of this project. Aides be comforted—there are many people who appreciate what you do and understand how special you are!

Speak Out!

If this book inspired you in your work and in your daily life, please help us spread the word. Our goal is to give every aide access to this wonderful book.

Special prices are available for organizations wishing to purchase multiple copies.

Single copy price	$12.95 plus $2 shipping

Copies Purchased	*Discounts*
2 to 10 copy price	25% off the single copy price, plus actual shipping
11 to 50 copy price	30% off ($9.07), plus actual shipping
51 to 100 copy price	35% off ($8.42), plus actual shipping
100+	40% off ($7.77), plus actual shipping

Single copy orders can be placed by mailing a check or money order to:

For Goodness' Sake
Hartman Publishing, Inc.
PO Box 91628
Albuquerque, NM 87199-1628

Multiple copy orders can be placed by phone with a credit card (Visa, MasterCard, or Discover) or by company purchase order.

Hartman Publishing, Inc.
Phone   505-291-1274
Fax   505-291-1284
hartmanonline.com

Thank you for spreading the word!

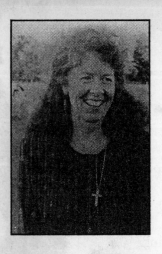

*B*ethany Knight lives at Shantivanam (peace forest), 130 acres of woods, meadows and ponds in northern Vermont, where she writes and leads workshops and retreats on spirituality, peacemaking and meaningful living.

She is a former long term care ombudsman, healthcare executive, lobbyist, newspaper reporter and gubernatorial speechwriter. Bethany is also a licensed pastor, nursing assistant and long term care insurance agent.

In December, 1998, she was a participant in the Way of Peace, a 54-person, international pilgrimage in India, led by the Dalai Lama.

A graduate of the University of Michigan and Central Michigan University, Bethany holds a BA in journalism and an MA in recreation and parks administration. She has done post graduate work at Duke Divinity School.

Bethany and her husband, Dr. Thurmond Knight, a maker of cellos, violins and violas, have two grown children, Chelsea and Elliot.